MRI of the Newborn, Part 2

Guest Editors

CLAUDIA M. HILLENBRAND, PhD
THIERRY A.G.M. HUISMAN, MD

MAGNETIC RESONANCE IMAGING CLINICS OF NORTH AMERICA

www.mri.theclinics.com

Consulting Editors
VIVIAN S. LEE, MD, PhD, MBA
LYNNE STEINBACH, MD
SURESH MUKHERJI, MD

February 2012 • Volume 20 • Number 1

SAUNDERS an imprint of ELSEVIER, Inc.

W.B. SAUNDERS COMPANY
A Division of Elsevier Inc.

1600 John F. Kennedy Boulevard ● Suite 1800 ● Philadelphia, Pennsylvania 19103-2899

http://www.theclinics.com

MRI CLINICS OF NORTH AMERICA Volume 20, Number 1
February 2012 ISSN 1064-9689, ISBN 13: 978-1-4557-3887-8

Editor: Barton Dudlick
Developmental Editor: Eva Kulig

Magnetic Resonance Imaging Clinics of North America (ISSN 1064-9689) is published quarterly by Elsevier Inc., 360 Park Avenue South, New York, NY 10010-1710. Months of issue are February, May, August, and November. Business and Editorial Offices: 1600 John F. Kennedy Blvd., Ste. 1800, Philadelphia, PA 19103-2899. Customer Service Office: 3251 Riverport Lane, Maryland Heights, MO 63043. Periodicals postage paid at New York, NY and additional mailing offices. Subscription prices are $337.00 per year (domestic individuals), $541.00 per year (domestic institutions), $172.00 per year (domestic students/residents), $376.00 per year (Canadian individuals), $678.00 per year (Canadian institutions), $488.00 per year (international individuals), $678.00 per year (international institutions), and $249.00 per year (international and Canadian students/residents). International air speed delivery is included in all *Clinics* subscription prices. All prices are subject to change without notice. **POSTMASTER:** Send address changes to *Magnetic Resonance Imaging Clinics*, Elsevier Health Sciences Division, Subscription Customer Service, 3251 Riverport Lane, Maryland Heights, MO 63043. Customer Service (orders, claims, online, change of address): Elsevier Health Sciences Division, Subscription Customer Service, 3251 Riverport Lane, Maryland Heights, MO 63043. Tel:1-800-654-2452 (U.S. and Canada); 314-447-8871 (outside U.S. and Canada). Fax: 314-447-8029. E-mail: journalscustomerservice-usa@elsevier.com (for print support); journalsonlinesupport-usa@elsevier.com (for online support).

Reprints. For copies of 100 or more of articles in this publication, please contact the Commercial Reprints Department, Elsevier Inc., 360 Park Avenue South, New York, NY 10010-1710. Tel.: 212-633-3812; Fax: 212-462-1935; E-mail: reprints@elsevier.com.

Magnetic Resonance Imaging Clinics of North America is covered in the *RSNA Index of Imaging Literature, MEDLINE/PubMed (Index Medicus),* and *EMBASE/Excerpta Medica.*

Printed in the United States of America.

GOAL STATEMENT

The goal of *Magnetic Resonance Imaging Clinics of North America* is to keep practicing physicians up to date with current clinical practice by providing timely articles reviewing the state of the art in patient care.

ACCREDITATION

The *Magnetic Resonance Imaging Clinics of North America* is planned and implemented in accordance with the Essential Areas and Policies of the Accreditation Council for Continuing Medical Education (ACCME) through the joint sponsorship of the University of Virginia School of Medicine and Elsevier. The University of Virginia School of Medicine is accredited by the ACCME to provide continuing medical education for physicians.

The University of Virginia School of Medicine designates this enduring material activity for a maximum of *15 AMA PRA Category 1 Credit*(s)™ for each issue, 60 credits per year. Physicians should claim only the credit commensurate with the extent of their participation in the activity.

The American Medical Association has determined that physicians not licensed in the US who participate in this CME enduring material activity are eligible for a maximum of *15 AMA PRA Category 1 Credit*(s)™ for each issue, 60 credits per year.

Credit can be earned by reading the text material, taking the CME examination online at http://www.theclinics.com/home/cme, and completing the evaluation. After taking the test, you will be required to review any and all incorrect answers. Following completion of the test and evaluation, your credit will be awarded and you may print your certificate.

FACULTY DISCLOSURE/CONFLICT OF INTEREST

The University of Virginia School of Medicine, as an ACCME accredited provider, endorses and strives to comply with the Accreditation Council for Continuing Medical Education (ACCME) Standards of Commercial Support, Commonwealth of Virginia statutes, University of Virginia policies and procedures, and associated federal and private regulations and guidelines on the need for disclosure and monitoring of proprietary and financial interests that may affect the scientific integrity and balance of content delivered in continuing medical education activities under our auspices.

The University of Virginia School of Medicine requires that all CME activities accredited through this institution be developed independently and be scientifically rigorous, balanced and objective in the presentation/discussion of its content, theories and practices.

All authors/editors participating in an accredited CME activity are expected to disclose to the readers relevant financial relationships with commercial entities occurring within the past 12 months (such as grants or research support, employee, consultant, stock holder, member of speakers bureau, etc.). The University of Virginia School of Medicine will employ appropriate mechanisms to resolve potential conflicts of interest to maintain the standards of fair and balanced education to the reader. Questions about specific strategies can be directed to the Office of Continuing Medical Education, University of Virginia School of Medicine, Charlottesville, Virginia.

The faculty and staff of the University of Virginia Office of Continuing Medical Education have no financial affiliations to disclose.

The authors/editors listed below have identified no professional or financial affiliations for themselves or their spouse/partner:
Sarah Barth, (Acquisitions Editor); Nancy Chauvin, MD; Alan Daneman, MD, FRCPC; Eduard de Lange, MD (Test Author); Philippe Demaerel, MD, PhD; Monica Epelman, MD; Andreia V. Faria, MD, PhD; Roxana S. Gunny, MBBS, FRCR; Claudia M. Hillenbrand, PhD; Thierry A.G.M. Huisman, MD, EQNR, FICIS; Vivian S. Lee, MD, PhD, MBA (Consulting Editor); Maarten H. Lequin, MD; Doris Lin, MD, PhD; Kenichi Oishi, MD, PhD; Andrea Rossi, MD; Paolo Tortori-Donati, MD; and Aphrodite Tzifa, MD, MRCPCH.

The authors/editors listed below identified the following professional or financial affiliations for themselves or their spouse/partner:
Wolfgang Hirsch, MD receives research funding from Bayer Vital GmbH.
Susumu Mori, PhD is co-founder of AnatomyWorks.
Suresh Mukherji, MD (Consulting Editor) is a consultant for Philips Medical Systems.
Reza Razavi, MD, FRCP is an industry funded research/investigator for Philips Healthcare.
Arne Reykowski, PhD is employed by Invivo Corporation.
Tobias Schaeffter, PhD is an industry funded research/investigator for Philips Healthcare.
Lynne Steinbach, MD (Consulting Editor) is a consultant for Pfizer, Inc.

Disclosure of Discussion of non-FDA approved uses for pharmaceutical products and/or medical devices:
The University of Virginia School of Medicine, as an ACCME provider, requires that all faculty presenters identify and disclose any "off label" uses for pharmaceutical and medical device products. The University of Virginia School of Medicine recommends that each physician fully review all the available data on new products or procedures prior to instituting them with patients.

TO ENROLL

To enroll in the Magnetic Resonance Imaging Clinics of North America Continuing Medical Education program, call customer service at 1-800-654-2452 or visit us online at www.theclinics.com/home/cme. The CME program is available to subscribers for an additional fee of $196.00.

Contributors

CONSULTING EDITORS

VIVIAN S. LEE, MD, PhD, MBA
Professor of Radiology, Physiology, and
Neurosciences; Vice-Dean for Science; Senior
Vice-President and Chief Scientific Officer at
New York University Langone Medical Center,
New York, New York

SURESH MUKHERJI, MD
Professor and Chief of Neuroradiology and
Head and Neck Radiology; Professor of
Radiology, Otolaryngology Head and Neck
Surgery, Radiation Oncology, Periodontics and
Oral Medicine, University of Michigan Health
System, Ann Arbor, Michigan

LYNNE STEINBACH, MD
Professor of Clinical Radiology and
Orthopaedic Surgery at the University
of California, San Francisco, San Francisco,
California

GUEST EDITORS

CLAUDIA M. HILLENBRAND, PhD
Assistant Member, Division of Translational
Imaging Research, Department of Radiological
Sciences, St Jude Children's Research
Hospital, Memphis, Tennessee

THIERRY A.G.M. HUISMAN, MD, EQNR, FICIS
Professor, Division of Pediatric Radiology,
Department of Radiology and Radiological
Science, Johns Hopkins Hospital, Baltimore,
Maryland

AUTHORS

NANCY CHAUVIN, MD
Assistant Professor of Radiology,
Department of Radiology, The Children's
Hospital of Philadelphia, Philadelphia,
Pennsylvania

ALAN DANEMAN, MD, FRCPC
Professor of Radiology, Department of
Diagnostic Imaging, The Hospital for Sick
Children, University of Toronto, Toronto,
Ontario, Canada

PHILIPPE DEMAEREL, MD, PhD
Department of Radiology, University Hospital
K.U. Leuven, Leuven, Belgium

MONICA EPELMAN, MD
Assistant Professor of Radiology, Director of
Neonatal Imaging, Department of Radiology,
The Children's Hospital of Philadelphia,
Philadelphia, Pennsylvania

ANDREIA V. FARIA, MD, PhD
Assistant Professor of Radiology, The Russell
H. Morgan Department of Radiology and
Radiological Science, The Johns Hopkins
University School of Medicine, Baltimore,
Maryland

ROXANA S. GUNNY, MBBS, MRCP, FRCR
Radiology Department, Great Ormond Street
Hospital and University College Hospital,
London, United Kingdom

CLAUDIA M. HILLENBRAND, PhD
Assistant Member, Division of Translational Imaging Research, Department of Radiological Sciences, St Jude Children's Research Hospital, Memphis, Tennessee

WOLFGANG HIRSCH, MD
Professor of Radiology, Universität Leipzig, Selbstständige Abteilung für Pädiatrische Radiologie, Leipzig, Germany

THIERRY A.G.M. HUISMAN, MD, EQNR, FICIS
Professor of Radiology and Radiological Science; Director, Division of Pediatric Radiology, Department of Radiology and Radiological Science, Johns Hopkins Hospital, Baltimore, Maryland

MAARTEN H. LEQUIN, MD
Department of Pediatric Radiology, Sophia Children's Hospital, University Hospital Rotterdam, GJ Rotterdam, The Netherlands

DORIS LIN, MD, PhD
Department of Radiology, John Hopkins Medical Center, Baltimore, Maryland

SUSUMU MORI, PhD
Professor of Radiology, The Russell H. Morgan Department of Radiology and Radiological Science, The Johns Hopkins University School of Medicine; F.M. Kirby Research Center for Functional Brain Imaging, Kennedy Krieger Institute, Baltimore, Maryland

KENICHI OISHI, MD, PhD
Assistant Professor of Radiology, The Russell H. Morgan Department of Radiology and Radiological Science, The Johns Hopkins University School of Medicine, Baltimore, Maryland

REZA RAZAVI, MD, FRCP
Professor of Paediatric Cardiovascular Sciences, Division of Imaging Sciences, King's College London BHF Centre, Rayne Institute, St Thomas' Hospital; Department of Paediatric Cardiology, Evelina Children's Hospital, Guy's and St Thomas' Hospital NHS Trust, London, United Kingdom

ARNE REYKOWSKI, PhD
Director, Research and Predevelopment, Invivo Corporation, Gainesville, Florida

ANDREA ROSSI, MD
Department of Pediatric Neuroradiology, G. Gaslini Children's Research Hospital, Genova, Italy

TOBIAS SCHAEFFTER, PhD
Philip Harris Chair in Imaging Sciences, Division of Imaging Sciences, King's College London BHF Centre, Rayne Institute, St Thomas' Hospital, Guy's and St Thomas' Hospital Trust, London, United Kingdom

PAOLO TORTORI-DONATI, MD
Department of Pediatric Neuroradiology, G. Gaslini Children's Research Hospital, Genova, Italy

APHRODITE TZIFA, MD, MRCPCH
Research Associate in Interventional MRI; Honorary Consultant Paediatric Cardiologist, Division of Imaging Sciences, King's College London BHF Centre, NIHR Biomedical Research Centre at Guy's and St Thomas' Hospital NHS Foundation Trust; Department of Paediatric Cardiology, Evelina Children's Hospital, Guy's & St Thomas' Hospital NHS Trust, London, United Kingdom

Contents

The main neonatal stroke syndromes discussed in this article are: arterial ischemic stroke (AIS), including perinatal AIS, and "presumed" perinatal AIS; cerebral venous thrombosis, including cortical vein and venous sinus thrombosis and germinal matrix hemorrhage/periventricular hemorrhagic infarction; and intraparenchymal hemorrhage. This review discusses general pathophysiological mechanisms and the role of imaging in these conditions.

Magnetic resonance (MR) imaging should be part of the routine workup in suspected inflicted brain injury. The inclusion of diffusion-weighted MR imaging is essential for assessment of acute hypoxic-ischemic brain injury because of its sensitivity to delineate the extent of the lesions and because of its prognostic significance. MR imaging may offer additional help in dating the intracranial hemorrhages, but a precise timing is often difficult if not impossible.

The development of the spinal canal and its contents is highly complex and involves multiple programmed anatomic and functional developmental and maturational processes. Correct and detailed knowledge about spinal malformations is essential to understand and recognize these lesions early (preferably prenatally) to counsel parents during pregnancy, to plan possible intrauterine treatments, and to make decisions about the mode of delivery and the immediate postnatal treatment. This article discusses the imaging findings of the most frequently encountered neonatal spinal malformations and correlates these findings with the relevant embryologic processes. The presented classification is based on a correlation of clinical, neuroradiologic, and embryologic data.

This article discusses neonatal magnetic resonance (MR) imaging and reviews equipment and procedures for MR-related transport, sedation, monitoring, and scanning. MR is gaining importance in the diagnosis and clinical management of critically ill, and often very low birth weight infants, so research is ongoing to make transport and examination safer and imaging more successful. Efforts are focused on integration of dedicated neonate MR scanners in neonatal intensive care units, improvements in incubator technology and handling, and more efficient use of scan/sedation time by choosing dedicated neonate coil arrays that improve the signal-to-noise-ratio and facilitate the choice of modern imaging techniques.

Magnetic Resonance Imaging Clinics of North America

THE CLINICS ARE NOW AVAILABLE ONLINE!

Access your subscription at:
www.theclinics.com

Preface

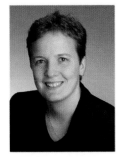
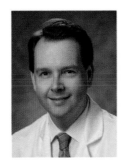

Claudia M. Hillenbrand, PhD   Thierry A.G.M. Huisman, MD, EQNR, FICIS

Guest Editors

This second issue dedicated to MRI of the newborn infant published in the series *Magnetic Resonance Imaging Clinics of North America* was believed necessary because MRI studies during the diagnostic workup of newborn infants not only are complex but also cover multiple groups of diseases and pathologies that may simultaneously involve various anatomical regions. This issue discusses the topics that could not be covered in the first issue.

The articles in this second issue are again written by teams of international experts that are well recognized for their contributions in their particular field of interest. In contrast to the first issue, the presented collection of articles not only discusses well-defined newborn pathologies (perinatal stroke, inflicted brain injury, spinal dysraphia) but also focuses on technical aspects of newborn imaging (technical perspectives of newborn imaging, advanced neonatal neuro-MRI). In addition, the competing or complementing role of head ultrasonography in relation to MRI is discussed. Finally, less frequently applied or used, but not less important, recent or technically challenging MRI developments and techniques (MR-guided cardiovascular interventions and postmortem MRI) are presented.

We are aware that the presented collection of articles in this two-issue edition on MRI of the newborn infant is far from complete. Many more indications for MRI are evolving; however, we are convinced that these articles will be helpful for every radiologist, neuroradiologist, pediatric radiologist, and whoever is interested in MR imaging of the newborn infant. With the current rapid development in the MR hard- and software, an expanded follow-up multi-issue edition may be necessary in a couple of years.

We hope that you will enjoy reading the articles as much as we have enjoyed working with the various authors. We again would like to express our special and sincere thanks to our expert friends who were willing to invest their time in preparing these articles. Finally, without the expert help of the Elsevier team, in particular, Barton Dudlick and Joanne Husovski, this project would not have been possible.

Last but not least, it has been a pleasure and honor for us to work as a MD-PhD team on this exciting topic.

Claudia M. Hillenbrand, PhD
Division of Translational Imaging Research
Department of Radiological Sciences
St Jude Children's Research Hospital
262 Danny Thomas Place
Memphis, TN 38105, USA

Thierry A.G.M. Huisman, MD, EQNR, FICIS
Division of Pediatric Radiology
Department of Radiology
and Radiological Science
Johns Hopkins Hospital
600 North Wolfe Street
Nelson, B-173
Baltimore, MD 21287-0842, USA

E-mail addresses:
claudia.hillenbrand@stjude.org (C.M. Hillenbrand)
thuisma1@jhmi.edu (T.A.G.M. Huisman)

Magn Reson Imaging Clin N Am 20 (2012) xi
doi:10.1016/j.mric.2011.11.001
1064-9689/12/$ – see front matter © 2012 Elsevier Inc. All rights reserved.

Imaging of Perinatal Stroke

Roxana S. Gunny, MBBS, MRCP, FRCR[a,b,]*, Doris Lin, MD, PhD[c]

KEYWORDS

- Perinatal arterial ischemic stroke
- Presumed perinatal arterial ischemic stroke
- Cerebral sinovenous thrombosis
- Cerebral venous thrombosis
- Germinal matrix hemorrhage-intraventricular hemorrhage
- Periventricular hemorrhagic infarction
- Intraparenchymal hemorrhage

The main neonatal stroke syndromes discussed in this review are: arterial ischemic stroke (AIS), including perinatal arterial ischemic stroke (PAIS) and "presumed" perinatal AIS; cerebral venous thrombosis (CVT), including cortical vein and venous sinus thrombosis and germinal matrix hemorrhage/periventricular hemorrhagic infarction; and intraparenchymal hemorrhage. Cerebral infarction in neonates may also occur as a result of cerebral hypotension causing hypoxic-ischemic brain injury, multiple vascular occlusions in meningoencephalitis and cerebritis, and in some rare congenital disorders such as incontinentia pigmenti. Infarctions due to abnormal metabolism at a cellular level may occur in neurometabolic disorders such as molybdenum cofactor deficiency, organic acidemias, and hypoglycemia. These other causes of cerebral infarction are beyond the scope of this article.

The World Health Organization defines stroke as "a clinical syndrome of rapidly developing focal or global disturbance of brain function lasting more than 24 hours or leading to death with no obvious nonvascular cause." This definition of stroke as a clinical syndrome with acute onset of a neurologic deficit is not readily applicable to strokes occurring in early life, either in children or in neonates. It is recognized that by this definition, children will have a nonvascular cause for their neurologic presentation in 1 out of 3 cases.[1]

Furthermore, neonates with an acute stroke may be asymptomatic, particularly preterm infants, or they may have a nonspecific clinical presentation such as lethargy, hypotonia, apnea, or feeding difficulties. The published series that have reported the highest rates of neonatal stroke are those in which the diagnosis was made by detecting an infarct on neuroimaging performed during routine screening rather than in symptomatic infants. For these reasons the diagnosis of stroke in neonates, as in children, relies on radiologic (or pathologic) confirmation.

It is also recognized that some strokes occur in utero before birth. In the published literature perinatal stroke has been inconsistently defined as a focal cerebrovascular insult sustained at any time between 20 and 28 gestational weeks and 7 to 28 days of neonatal life. In an attempt to reach some consensus of definition, at least for the purposes of research, the National Institute of Child Health-National Institute of Neurological Disorders and Stroke (NICH-NINDS) perinatal workshop defined perinatal stroke as a "a group of heterogeneous conditions in which there is focal disruption of cerebral blood flow secondary to arterial or cerebral venous thrombus or embolization" occurring "between 20 weeks of fetal life through the 28th postnatal day and confirmed by neuroimaging or neuropathological studies."[2] Their imaging criteria defined stroke as either

[a] Radiology Department, Great Ormond Street Hospital, Great Ormond Street, London WC1N 3JH, UK
[b] Radiology Department, University College Hospital, London, UK
[c] Department of Radiology, John Hopkins Medical Center, Baltimore, MD, USA
* Corresponding author. Radiology Department, Great Ormond Street Hospital, Great Ormond Street, London WC1N 3JH, UK.
E-mail address: roxana.gunny@gosh.nhs.uk

Magn Reson Imaging Clin N Am 20 (2012) 1–33
doi:10.1016/j.mric.2011.10.001

a partial or complete occlusion of a vessel with a focal brain lesion in that territory or brain imaging corresponding to infarction in a recognized vascular territory. By this definition an acute neurologic presentation is no longer necessary, while neuroimaging has become essential in making the diagnosis of perinatal stroke.

Some children in whom stroke is not detected in the neonatal period may present later with signs such as asymmetry of reach and grasp, failure to reach normal milestones, postnatal seizures, and congenital hemiplegia. In these children, in whom the presentation of hemiplegia or seizures is not acute, the diagnosis of presumed perinatal AIS is made based on neuroimaging appearances of a chronic arterial territory infarct. Hence the timing of the AIS is remote from the clinical presentation. It is assumed to be perinatal on the basis that beyond the neonatal period, stroke is likely to have presented as an acute focal or global neurologic deficit, and also on the presence of characteristic imaging features that establish that the stroke most likely occurred in early life.

The NICH-NINDS classification separates perinatal stroke into 3 groups: (1) fetal ischemic stroke diagnosed before birth using imaging or in stillborns on the basis of postmortem pathologic examination, (2) neonatal ischemic stroke diagnosed after birth and before the 28th postnatal day (including preterm infants), and (3) presumed perinatal ischemic stroke, diagnosed in infants older than 28 days in whom it is presumed (but not certain) that the ischemic event occurred sometime between the 20th week of fetal life through the 28th postnatal day.[2]

Cranial ultrasonography, computed tomography (CT), and magnetic resonance (MR) imaging are the 3 main imaging techniques available to image the neonatal brain. Ultrasonography is readily available, inexpensive, portable, and can be performed at the bedside. It is usually the first-line brain-imaging technique performed on the neonatal unit, and allows serial examinations to be performed without transfer of the sick neonate to the radiology department. However, ultrasonography lacks sensitivity for all types of neonatal stroke, particularly lesions at interfaces with bone such as posterior fossa lesions and peripherally based cortical lesions. It is dependent on the level of skill and experience of the operator. CT has some advantages over MR imaging in that it is a quicker examination with less need for sedation. CT depicts venous sinus thrombosis and hemorrhage well. However, potential concerns regarding radiation effects on the developing neonatal brain[3] and increased lifelong risk of cancer[4] limit its use to neonates who are acutely deteriorating clinically

and in whom neurosurgical intervention is being considered, or when there is limited access or contraindication to MR imaging. Multislice brain CT should be performed according to low-dose pediatric protocols that vary dose according to weight and age. The authors do not recommend the use of currently commercially available portable CT scanners for imaging the neonatal or infant brain because diagnostic quality is less good and a greater radiation dose is required compared with departmental scanners. Overall, CT is less sensitive for the detection and characterization of brain lesions, and MR imaging is the modality of choice for evaluating the neonatal brain. However, it is important that MR imaging and sedation protocols are optimized to allow multiplanar imaging, multiple sequences (T1, T2, and diffusion-weighted imaging) providing differing tissue contrasts, and vascular imaging (MR angiography, MR venography) without artifacts from motion.

PERINATAL ARTERIAL ISCHEMIC STROKE
Incidence

Eighty percent of perinatal stroke is attributable to AIS; this differs from the relative incidence of AIS in children in whom ischemic stroke (AIS and cerebral sinovenous thrombosis [CSVT]) and hemorrhagic stroke occur with the same frequency. The incidence of perinatal AIS is estimated to occur in around 1 in 1600 to 5000 births in populations from the United Kingdom, Switzerland, the United States, and Estonia.[5–8] The United Kingdom study found that acute PAIS was more common in boys than in girls whereas presumed PAIS was more common in girls.[5]

These variations in incidence may be explained by differing diagnostic criteria and use of MR imaging, as well as different study populations. For example, the Estonian study included all neonatal stroke, including hemorrhagic stroke, in its cohort. Both this and the United States study included retrospectively diagnosed, presumed PAIS as well as neonatal AIS. These two studies had the highest incidences and showed that many perinatal strokes (42%,[7] 68%[8] of all PAIS) are not diagnosed until later in life. This figure may still be an underestimate of the true incidence of PAIS, as it is likely that some PAIS is asymptomatic or associated with very mild deficits and therefore may go undetected during life. A hospital-based study by Benders and colleagues[9] found that PAIS is not uncommon in preterm infants under gestational age of approximately 34 weeks, with an even greater incidence of 7 in 1000. Two possible explanations for this relatively high incidence may be the use of routine cranial ultrasonography in this population and their exposure to more invasive procedures during their stay in the neonatal intensive care unit.

Perinatal stroke affects 20 to 62.5 per 100,000 live births. This high incidence compares with an annual incidence rate of stroke in children after the first month of life of 2.3 to 13 per 100,000 per year, similar to the incidence of pediatric brain tumor. The peak incidence of AIS is in the first year of life, and does not rise to these levels again until much later in life.[10] The risk is highest in the perinatal period soon before birth and in the month after. This increased risk of neonatal AIS is mirrored by a parallel increased risk of ischemic stroke in the mother that is up to 5 times greater just before and for the day after delivery than earlier in pregnancy or when not pregnant.[11] This increased maternal and neonatal risk of ischemic stroke is related to the activation of coagulation cascades during normal birth, likely to be an evolutionary adaptation to reduce the risk of blood loss during delivery.

Pathophysiology and Risk Factors

The majority of PAIS is most likely to be caused by thromboembolism passing from the placenta through the patent neonatal foramen ovale, although other potential sources include the fetal/neonatal heart and extracranial vessels (**Box 1** and **Fig. 1**). By the end of the embryonic period the developing cerebral arterial system is already similar anatomically to that of the adult, and therefore the arterial territories that are affected in PAIS are the same as those in adults. Most PAIS occurs in the middle cerebral artery (MCA) territory, typically either a complete MCA infarct or a posterior truncal infarct, and the left MCA is affected 3 to 4 times more commonly than the right.[12] This bias has been explained as the result of hemodynamic arterial flow; placental emboli or systemic venous emboli in the fetus or neonate may pass through a patent foramen ovale or patent ductus arteriosus directly into the left common carotid artery and hence to the left MCA. The sick newborn is also at risk from right-to-left shunting associated with respiratory disease, pulmonary hypertension, or congenital heart disease.

Hence most of the associated risk factors for perinatal stroke appear to be related to an increased propensity for thromboembolism. The physiologic activation of the coagulation cascade in the fetus and mother around delivery is normally a transient phenomenon, which may explain why the recurrence risk of neonatal stroke is extremely low, and then mainly seems to recur in children in whom there is an underlying procoagulation

Box 1
Risk factors for perinatal stroke

Maternal factors

　Autoimmune disorders

　Coagulation disorders (Protein C deficiency, Protein S deficiency, Factor V Leiden)

　Anticardiolipin antibodies

　Twin-to-twin transfusion syndrome

　In utero cocaine exposure

　Infection

Placental factors

　Placental thrombosis

　Placental abruption

　Placental infection

　Fetomaternal hemorrhage

Cardiac disorders

　Congenital heart disease

　Patent ductus arteriosus

　Pulmonary valve atresia

　Cardiac surgery (associated with cardiac bypass, atrial balloon septostomy)

Fetal and neonatal blood and lipid disorders

　Polycythemia

　Disseminated intravascular coagulopathy

　Factor V Leiden mutation

　Protein S deficiency

　Protein C deficiency

　Prothrombin mutation

　Homocysteine

　Lipoprotein(a)

　Factor VIII

Infection

　Central nervous system infection

　Systemic infection

Vasculopathy

　Vascular malformation or defect

Trauma and catheterization

Birth asphyxia

Dehydration

Extracorporeal membrane oxygenation

Modified from Nelson KB, Lynch JK. Stroke in newborn infants [review]. Lancet Neurol 2004;3: 150–8; with permission.

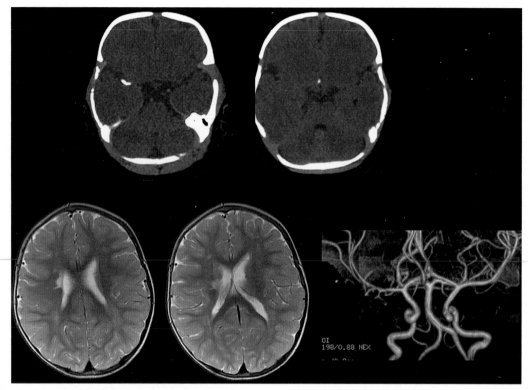

Fig. 1. A 3-year-old child referred to the authors, born at 34 weeks and presenting with left hemplegia. (*Top row*) CT at 1 month of age shows already calcified thrombus within the proximal right middle cerebral artery (MCA) and anterior cerebral artery (ACA). (*Bottom row*) Follow-up imaging at 3 years shows a mature right lenticulostriate infarct including head of caudate nucleus. Maximum-intensity projection of time-of-flight MR angiography shows attenuated flow within the right M1 and M2 segments.

defect.[13] This situation differs from that in AIS in children, in whom the recurrence risk is 6% to 13% with an even higher recurrence risk of transient ischemic attack (TIA) or "silent infarct."[14]

While thromboembolism is also a risk factor in pediatric stroke, it appears there is a greater range of underlying etiological factors for stroke in children; arteriopathy is one of the commonest causes of childhood stroke[15–17] and is associated with recurrence risk, a feature that has not been recognized (or systematically studied) in neonatal stroke. Beyond a few case reports in which the diagnosis of dissection was presumptive and made without pathognomonic radiological evidence of a dissection flap or intramural thrombus,[18] there is little evidence that arterial dissection is a common cause of PAIS, unlike in older children.[19]

Risk factors for thromboembolism for PAIS include fetal/neonatal, maternal, and placental factors, and are found in 42% to 78% of PAIS.[20] In one study thromboembolic risk factors were found in 68% of PAIS compared with 24% of normal controls.[21] Multiple risk factors for thromboembolism may coexist. Normal neonates already have several risk factors for thrombus formation in the perinatal period, including a raised hematocrit, presence of fetal hemoglobin, high procoagulant proteins, and increased blood viscosity.[10] Additional blood and lipid disorders are also associated with PAIS. Twin pregnancies have a greater risk of PAIS, which appears to be independent of twin-twin transfusion syndrome or co-twin demise.[22,23]

Congenital heart disease is an independent risk factor for perinatal stroke. White matter lesions are more common than arterial territory cortical infarcts. In studies investigating brain MR imaging abnormalities in children with congenital heart disease, periventricular white matter injury was seen on MR imaging in 16% to 43% of patients with congenital heart disease prior to any operative procedure.[24–26] The changes were focal and asymptomatic, and were seen in children without any acute postnatal hypoxic-ischemic event. Although established lesions do not appear to progress postoperatively, additional ischemic lesions are found after cardiac surgery.[27] Impairment of brain development during the fetal period in children with congenital heart disease (measured by quantitative advanced MR imaging techniques) is recognized.[28] It is suggested that the brains of children with congenital heart disease are immature and behave in a similar way to the brains of preterm babies affected by hypoxic-ischemic injury, and that the white matter is particularly susceptible. In these studies risk factors associated with acquired postoperative brain injury included risk factors for cerebral hypotension, such as cardiopulmonary bypass (CPB) with regional cerebral hypoperfusion, lower intraoperative cerebral hemoglobin oxygen saturation during the myocardial ischemic period of CPB, and low mean blood pressure during the first postoperative day.[25] However, neonates with congenital heart disease are also at risk of AIS. Preoperative AIS is typically arterial territory branch cortical infarction and is associated with balloon atrial septostomy, whereas white matter injury is not.[29] Children are also at risk of thromboembolic AIS from cardiac catheters and other vascular catheters. Extracorporeal membranous oxygenation (ECMO) is a specific thromboembolic risk. Specific artificial devices such as the Berlin Heart, a pediatric mechanical ventricular assist device, are also associated with neonatal AIS (**Fig. 2**).

Although an association with hypoxic-ischemic encephalopathy (HIE) in term babies has been described,[10,30] there is actually little evidence for HIE as a cause when strict diagnostic definitions are used.[31] The more usual scenario is a term baby born in good condition after an uncomplicated pregnancy and labor or elective cesarean section. Hypoglycemia is recognized as an independent risk factor for PAIS in preterm babies but not in term babies, in whom hypoglycemic brain injury usually manifests as bilateral parieto-occipital lobe infarction.

The placenta itself has an important role in the etiology of thromboembolism in perinatal stroke; placental disorders include thrombosis, abruption and fetomaternal hemorrhage, placental infection, and chorioamnionitis.[32] Placental thrombotic vasculopathy is a commonly recognized finding, and may be linked to maternal prothrombotic conditions. Emboli may also arise from umbilical vascular catheters.

Maternal factors associated with PAIS include maternal procoagulation tendencies and autoimmune disorders. Factor V Leiden deficiency, increased lipoprotein(a) and antiphospholipid antibodies, and heterozygosity or homozygosity of methyltetrahydrofolate reductase mutations are seen with greater frequency in neonates with PAIS and their mothers. Other maternal factors include a history of infertility, infection, preeclampsia, maternal trauma, diabetes, in utero cocaine use, prolonged labor, and instrumented delivery.[33] Primiparity has been identified as a risk factor in 30% to 75% of cases of PAIS in term infants but not in preterms. This finding may be more closely related to a prolonged second stage of labor, as primiparity did not remain a statistically significant independent risk factor on multivariate analysis.[7]

Clinical Presentation

Acute presentation in the neonatal period

Although epidemiologic data may be less accurate given the limitations of missed or later diagnoses, approximately 60% of cases of PAIS do present acutely in the neonatal period, mostly with recurrent focal seizures in the first 3 days of life.

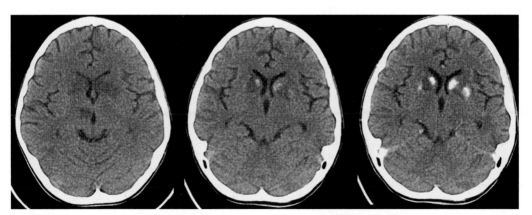

Fig. 2. CT brain scans of a 5-week-old baby with congenital heart disease presenting with seizures, who had received a Berlin Heart ventricular assist device and was therefore unable to have MR imaging. Unenhanced CT brain scans (*left, middle*) show bilateral low-density lesions in the basal ganglia and right thalamus in keeping with arterial perforator territory infarcts, with some hyperdensity due to secondary hemorrhagic transformation. Contrast was also given (*right*), showing enhancement in the regions of hemorrhagic transformation indicating disruption of the blood-brain barrier.

Therefore about 40% of the children do not have specific symptoms in the neonatal period, and are only recognized later with the emergence of motor impairment, developmental delay, specific cognitive deficiency, or seizures.[20] Twenty-five% to 40% of term infants with PAIS present with seizures.[10] After hypoxic ischemia, perinatal arterial ischemic stroke is the second most common cause of neonatal seizures in term newborns[34]; this differs from AIS in childhood whereby the most common presentations are an acute focal deficit (91%), seizures (23%), or headache (44%).

Typically PAIS occurs in a term baby with a normal antenatal course who appears generally well. The baby usually has a normal neurologic examination with preserved primitive reflexes, and no or minimal signs of encephalopathy. Usually the seizures in PAIS are focal with clinical recovery in between, matched by electroencephalography (EEG) changes of focal spikes and/or sharp waves during seizures, but usually a normal background EEG.[31] In other neonates there may be subtle, nonspecific neurologic signs of hypotonia, lethargy, poor feeding, duskiness, or apnea. Hemiparesis is rarely found on neurologic examination at this age. Hence the diagnosis of PAIS is made only when neuroimaging confirms a lesion consistent with focal infarction in an arterial vascular territory.

Presumed diagnosis of PAIS made retrospectively

Infants and children with presumed PAIS are diagnosed after the neonatal period; they do not have clinical signs during the neonatal period or may have signs that are so subtle that they escape detection. Such patients may present later with hemiplegia, focal hand weakness, or pathologic early hand preference occurring when younger than 1 year of age. These motor deficits are usually only detected from the middle of the first year of life onward, when coordinated voluntary motor activity is developing. Children may present with other long-term neurologic problems such as cognitive impairment and seizures.[35–39] In these children the diagnosis is presumptive, and relies on confirmation of neuroimaging findings of a chronic arterial territory infarct.

Fetal or preterm ischemic stroke

Fetuses may be diagnosed with AIS based on a routine early second-trimester anomaly screening ultrasound scan (ideally confirmed by MR imaging), on ultrasound scans done later in pregnancy for other reasons, or on postmortem examination. PAIS in preterm infants is more likely to be asymptomatic than in term babies, and is often detected as the result of routine cranial ultrasonography or brain MR imaging in the (sick) preterm infant. In one study PAIS was detected in 10% of all preterms who had routine cranial ultrasonography as part of their assessment. Equally PAIS was found in 10% of preterms who were symptomatic with apneas that were subsequently confirmed as seizures using amplitude-integrated EEG.[9]

Imaging

The role of imaging is to make or confirm the diagnosis of PAIS and to exclude stroke mimics such as encephalitis, hypoglycemia, and hypoxic ischemia. Neuroimaging can be used to help time the onset of the infarct and to confer information regarding prognosis. Neuroimaging definition criteria for PAIS are: (1) imaging evidence of a partial or complete occlusion of an artery in relation to a focal brain lesion, or (2) distribution of parenchymal lesion(s) that can only be explained by occlusion of a specific brain artery.[40]

Site

The developing arterial system is already similar to the mature arterial system by the end of the embryonic period, the major differences being in the watershed sites between arterial territories, which have shifted from the germinal matrix and periventricular regions to more lateral parasagittal cortex by term. Hence the lesion pattern caused by occlusion of a particular artery is already established by 20 gestational weeks and is consistent throughout life.

Any arterial territory may be involved; however, most infants with PAIS show involvement of the MCA territory (75%) and usually of the left hemisphere (55%). Posterior circulation infarction is relatively unusual, and this is comparable with the distribution in children in whom isolated anterior circulation infarcts (73%) are much more common than posterior circulation infarcts (21%). Multiple arterial territories may be involved in thromboembolic disease, and 6% to 25% of perinatal arterial ischemic strokes are bilateral. The most common MCA branches affected in term infants are the main branch of the MCA, resulting in complete MCA territory infarction, and the posterior MCA trunk, causing posterior temporal and parietal lobe infarction. After this, in decreasing order of frequency, are infarcts in the territories of the internal carotid, anterior cerebral, posterior cerebral, posterior communicating, and anterior choroidal arteries.[40,41] As in the term population, the majority of strokes in preterm infants involve the MCA (81%); however, the involvement of different branches of the MCA appears to change with gestational age. Involvement of one or more lenticulostriate branches was most common among infants with a gestational age of 28 to 32 weeks.[41]

Evolution of infarction on neuroimaging

Magnetic resonance imaging Swelling of astrocytes is seen on pathologic studies within 30 minutes of onset of ischemia, and by 4 to 6 hours swelling of oligodendrocyte nuclei and cytoplasm is seen microscopically.[42] MR imaging, particularly diffusion-weighted imaging, is more sensitive than both cranial ultrasonography and CT for the detection of acute AIS, and MR imaging is the modality of choice in the neuroimaging evaluation of suspected neonatal stroke.

Animal experiments show restricted diffusion on brain MR imaging scans within the infarcted parenchyma minutes after ischemia.[43] The exact mechanism accounting for the appearances of restricted diffusion in acute ischemia is not completely understood. In tissue ischemia energy depletion leads to disruption of the energy-dependent ion pump, which causes increased intracellular sodium and water and results in cytotoxic edema. There is a net shift of water from the extracellular space to the intracellular space, with reduced free water movement within the interstitial fluid. This shift is not the only contribution to the signal hyperintensity on diffusion-weighted images, as increased signal due to T2 effects becomes more important later when cytotoxic edema has already occurred.

On diffusion-weighted imaging the earliest changes of infarction are seen as signal hyperintensity in the affected arterial territory, and can be seen before changes on T2-weighted sequences are appreciated. The signal hyperintensity is maximal until 4 days after birth and slowly declines, but remains higher than in normal brain for up to 1 to 2 weeks.[44–46] These earliest diffusion-weighted signal hyperintensity changes are matched by low signal on calculated apparent diffusion coefficient (ADC) maps. The ADC values in infarction progressively decrease over the first 3 days before beginning to increase again, reaching normal values, or pseudonormalization, by 4 to 10 days.[47,48] It is suggested that this ADC change broadly correlates with the presence of cytotoxic edema. Thereafter, ADC values progressively increase as vasogenic edema develops. The evolution of these changes with time is probably similar to those changes described in adults though has not been systematically studied. However, the signal hyperintensity seen on diffusion-weighted images in adults often persists for longer, often appearing hyperintense weeks after the initial event. In adults the cortical gray matter shows a smaller drop in measured ADC values and a slightly faster rate of increase in ADC than white matter, hence pseudonormalization occurs slightly earlier in the cortical gray matter.[49] This appearance is also probably similar in neonates.

The cortex in the region of infarction is initially hyperintense on T2-weighted imaging for the first 6 days. It is seen as loss of the normal, relatively darker signal of the cortical ribbon in comparison with the unmyelinated white matter (**Fig. 3**). On T1 weighted imaging the cortex may appear relatively dark with respect to normal cortex. During this time the white matter also appears hyperintense on T2-weighted imaging, and this persists for 2 to 3 weeks or so before declining to eventually appear similar to unaffected brain. The white matter appears mildly hyperintense on T1-weighted imaging during the first 8 to 9 days compared with the normal cerebral white matter (though not as bright as the T1 shortening seen with subsequent haemorrhagic transformation or cortical highlighting). This feature is particularly apparent in acute neonatal AIS, possibly because of the relatively greater contrast between the normal low signal of the neonatal unmyelinated cerebral white matter and adjacent cortex.

Neonates have smaller vessels with lower blood flow velocities than children or adults, making MR angiography and MR venography of the neonatal brain more technically challenging for assessment of the vascular anatomy, vessel diameter, and flow. Three techniques are available: time-of-flight, phase-contrast, and contrast-enhanced MR angiography. Each has its advantages and disadvantages, but the first 2 techniques may be successfully used in the neonate without the need for contrast. In PAIS, MR angiography may show medium-vessel or large-vessel occlusion, supporting the pathogenesis of thromboembolism (**Fig. 4**), but may also be normal.

Ultrasonography Although relatively insensitive for the diagnosis of AIS, cranial ultrasonography is usually the first neuroimaging test that will be performed, either in symptomatic term infants or on routine screening of sick preterm infants. The typical appearances are a well-defined wedge-shaped region of increased echogenicity affecting cortex and white matter in a recognized arterial territory. Doppler studies in MCA infarcts may, or may not,[50] show transient reduced flow and pulsatility on the affected side that becomes similar to the contralateral unaffected side by 24 hours.[51] The exact reason for this is not known; possible explanations for the subsequent improved flow include migration of arterial embolus and

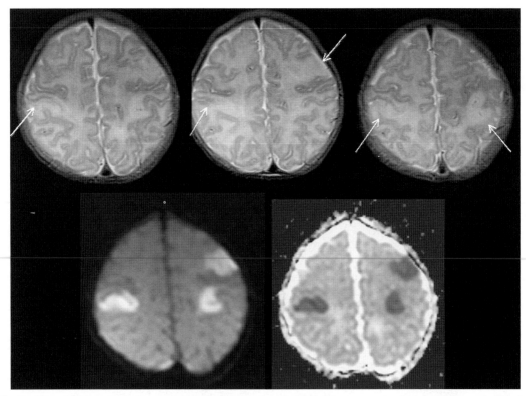

Fig. 3. MR axial T2-weighted images (*top row*), diffusion-weighted image, and calculated apparent diffusion coefficient (ADC) map (*bottom row*) of a term baby boy whose mother noticed jerking movements of his right limbs at 6 hours of life resolving within 20 minutes. While on the neonatal unit the baby again developed jerking movements of the right upper and lower limbs. Electroencephalography (EEG) showed left-sided focal seizures. MR imaging on day 3 of life showed bilateral multiple acute cortical branch MCA territory infarcts. Note the cortical and white matter signal hyperintensity on T2-weighted images with loss of normal cortical ribbon in some regions (*arrows*). The diffusion-weighted imaging increases the conspicuity of the lesions; these show restricted diffusion with signal hyperintensity on the diffusion-weighted image (*left*) matched by low signal on the ADC map (*right*).

compensatory cross-flow. Most neonatal strokes have a patent MCA by the time of presentation.

The sensitivity of ultrasonography for the detection of AIS increases with the age of the infarct (68% sensitive in the first 3 days compared with 87% between days 4 and 10[52]) but it is well recognized to miss small, peripherally located cortical infarcts, and posterior circulation infarcts, even when these are retrospectively diagnosed following a positive MR imaging study. Repeated imaging may be required to detect a lesion. Typically an MCA infarct is easier to diagnose when mass effect is at its greatest, around the third day, where ultrasonography may have some advantage over MR imaging is in the detection of small perforator territory AIS such as those seen in preterm infants.[9]

Necrosis and organization From 6 hours to 6 days coagulation necrosis is associated with damage to

the endothelium and breakdown of the blood-brain barrier, leading to vasogenic edema and brain swelling. Swelling of the affected brain is usually maximal at 3 days and is evidenced by sulcal effacement, and in large anterior circulation infarcts by subfalcine and uncal herniation with shift of midline structures. If the cerebral swelling progresses, contralateral hydrocephalus may develop. Although not routinely given, contrast enhancement may be seen as a consequence of disruption of the blood-brain barrier. Hemorrhage may be seen as the result of reperfusion of the infarct. Increased flow velocities such as diastolic arterial flow with a lowered resistance index and increased venous flow may be seen on ultrasonography as a result of regional luxury perfusion.

The pathologic description of laminar necrosis is of necrosis in the cortex; this may affect all layers or just the middle to deeper cortical layers (pseudolaminar necrosis). The imaging correlate of this is

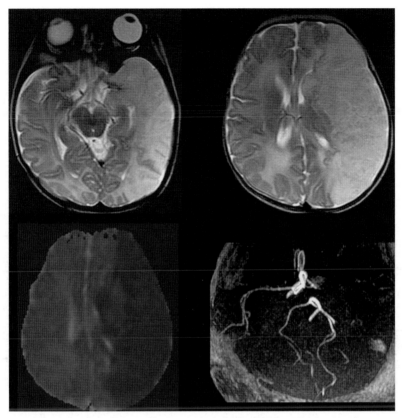

Fig. 4. A neonate presenting with focal seizures scanned on day 4 of life, with a large infarct involving the entire left MCA territory and anterior choroidal artery territory (anteromesial temporal lobe). Axial T2-weighted images (*top row*) show signal hyperintensity in the cortex and white matter with loss of the normal cortical ribbon and sulcal effacement, with some shift of midline structures to the right. There is some uncal herniation but no evidence of secondary infarction in the left posterior cerebral artery territory. ADC map (*bottom left*) shows restricted diffusion, and time-of-flight MR angiography (*bottom right*) shows absent flow in the left terminal carotid artery and left MCA. Cross-flow via the anterior communicating artery supplies the left ACA territory.

believed to be cortical highlighting, or T1 shortening localized to the cortex. This is seen from days 5 to 6 after onset; from this time the cortex also becomes dark on T2-weighted imaging These cortical changes are generally thought to be related to petechial hemorrhage or increased paramagnetic substances, release of myelin lipids, or calcification.[53,54] Susceptibility-weighted imaging has been used in attempts to differentiate the changes seen on T1-weighted imaging from hemorrhage; in one study the cortical highlighting did not correspond with dark signal on susceptibility imaging, and the assumption was made that the changes are not due to hemorrhage.[55] However, this study did not differentiate extracellular met as in methemoglobin hemoglobin, which is bright on both T1-weighted and T2-weighted sequences, from the other molecular forms of hemorrhage that do demonstrate susceptibility effects.

From 3 days to 6 weeks the infarct organizes, a process in which central liquefaction develops in necrotic areas with gliosis, breakdown of myelin, microcyst formation, calcification, and peripheral neovascularization. During this time the infarct shows signal changes in keeping with increased water content compared with unaffected brain, but has not yet cavitated. Strands of tissue may be seen crossing the infarct.

Tissue loss Cystic cavitation and atrophy in the affected arterial territory are seen from approximately 4 weeks after onset. Typically the cyst is lined by a gliotic scar, and there may be hemosiderin. On MR imaging this is seen as regions of cystic cavitation or encephalomalacia with surrounding signal change in keeping with gliosis. When imaged later in life, as in a presumed large perinatal MCA infarct the whole of the cerebral hemisphere appears smaller, and there may be compensatory expansion of the calvarial diploic space and paranasal and mastoid sinuses **(Fig. 5)**.

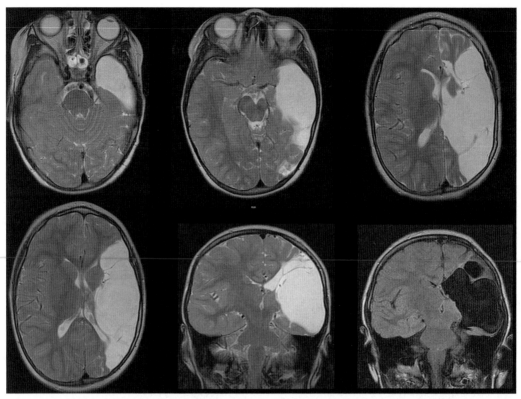

Fig. 5. A 5-year-old girl with long-standing right hemiplegia and intractable epilepsy secondary to a left sided infarct, considered for functional hemispherectomy in the authors' epilepsy surgery program. Note the large area of cystic cavitation in the left temporal, frontal, and parietal lobes in extended left MCA territory (with some additional anterior choroidal involvement as in the previous case, and atrophy of the left thalamus). The left hemicranium is smaller, and there is some expansion of the left calvarial diploic space. There is 3-site involvement of the basal ganglia, superficial cortex, and posterior limb of the internal capsule. There is imaging evidence of Wallerian degeneration with atrophy, and signal hyperintensity suggestive of gliosis in the ventral midbrain and pons.

Acute secondary neuronal pre-Wallerian and Wallerian degeneration Secondary signal intensity changes remote from the infarction are seen in the brainstem and thalamus in the first week. In some MCA infarcts, restricted diffusion occurs outside the MCA territory within the more caudal ipsilateral corticospinal tract within the brainstem (**Fig. 6**). These diffusion changes occur earlier than the signal hyperintensity on T2-weighted images and focal swelling seen subsequently. Within a few weeks these changes progress to mature injury with evidence of atrophy and gliosis, sometimes with T1 shortening, as a secondary neuronal degenerative or Wallerian-type phenomenon. Similarly, acute changes of restricted diffusion with subsequent T2 signal changes and swelling are also seen within the medial thalamus, which are likely attributable to secondary degeneration of corticothalamic projections. Contralateral cerebellar hemisphere atrophy may be seen as a result of crossed cerebellar diaschisis following MCA infarction.

Treatment

Although there are currently 3 international evidence-based stroke guidelines for the investigation and management of stroke in children, only the American Heart Association (AHA) Stroke Council guideline (2008) specifically addresses neonatal stroke.[56] There is no specific treatment for stroke, and management is supportive and directed at modification of etiological factors as well as treatment of the complications of stroke such as epilepsy. Recommendations for surgery are ventricular drainage of hydrocephalus complicating hematoma evacuation or shunting if hydrocephalus persists (Class I recommendation), and hematoma evacuation in the presence of raised intracranial pressure, though this may not necessarily improve outcome (Class II recommendation). Anticoagulation may be considered for recurrent thromboembolic stroke, but specific recommendations are not made. Thrombolytic agents are not recommended in neonates while

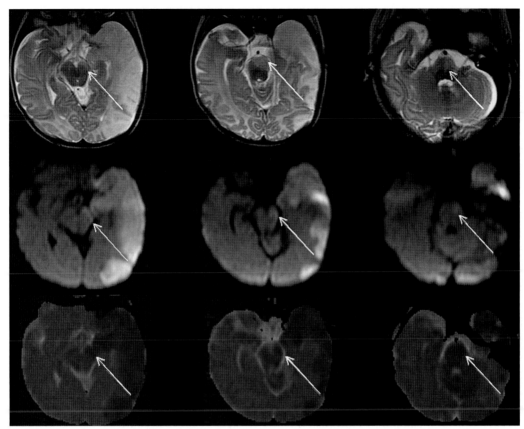

Fig. 6. A neonate with extended large MCA and anterior choroidal infarcts secondary to left terminal internal carotid artery occlusion scanned at day 5. Acute secondary neuronal degeneration of the corticospinal tract caudal to the MCA infarct (*arrows*). Axial T2-weighted images (*top row*) show signal hyperintensity within the left corticospinal tract affecting the left crus cerebri of the midbrain and left ventral pons. Diffusion-weighted images (*middle row*) and ADC maps (*lower row*) show restricted diffusion (low signal on ADC maps, high signal on diffusion-weighted imaging).

more information about the safety and effectiveness of these agents is awaited.

Predicting Outcome

The main adverse outcomes following PAIS are hemiplegia, epilepsy, visual impairment, cognitive impairment, and behavioral difficulties. However, some children (33%–40%) will have a normal outcome,[57,58] presumably due to plasticity of the neonatal brain.[59] There is no evidence of an increased risk of death in neonates with AIS unless there are additional complicating factors such as congenital heart disease or HIE. All of the outcome studies to date show that the outcome for babies with stroke is better than that for older children and adults.

Motor Impairment

Up to 50% of neonates with PAIS will develop subsequent hemiplegia. Hemiplegia is usually not evident in the neonate or infant, but may be

detected in later life. Children with PAIS may also develop more subtle motor impairments, which may present even later. Nevertheless, most children will still be able to achieve independent walking. Early MR imaging performed around the time of the acute infarct can be used to predict the subsequent development of hemiplegia. In general, small infarcts of the posterior cortical branches of the MCA or posterior cerebral artery are associated with a better prognosis than large main-branch MCA infarcts. Involvement of 3 sites of cerebral infarction (basal ganglia, posterior limb of the internal capsule, and temporoparietal cortical infarction) as seen in main-branch MCA infarction predicts future hemiplegia, whether occurring at term or preterm.[20,38,60] Acute pre-Wallerian secondary neuronal degeneration with restricted diffusion in the corticospinal tract caudal to the infarct also predicts future hemiplegia.[61] Combining these findings further refines motor outcome prediction. In their study of 73 infants with PAIS affecting the MCA territory, Husson and colleagues found that 72% of babies with superficial cortex, basal ganglia involvement, and restricted diffusion of the corticospinal tract (CST) developed later motor impairment by age 2 years.[62] Mixed infarctions involving superficial cortex and basal ganglia (P<.001) and CST involvement (P<.001) were highly predictive of hemiplegia, whereas most babies (88%) with isolated superficial cortical infarcts did not develop future motor impairment. Absence of CST involvement predicted normal motor outcome in 94%.

The risk of epilepsy for a child with PAIS increases with time, and PAIS is a common cause of epilepsy in children referred for consideration of epilepsy surgery. Epilepsy may be seen in up to 50% of children, whereas cognitive outcome is more frequently impaired in PAIS than in childhood stroke, and ranges from 25% to 40%. However, the success of early brain MR imaging in predicting subsequent epilepsy, cognitive outcome, and behavioral difficulties is more limited.[63] Some studies suggest that cognitive impairment is worse when there are more extensive main-branch infarcts involving superficial cortex and deep gray matter.[20,64] Other studies suggest that cognitive outcome is more closely associated with hemiplegia and epilepsy than extent of MCA lesion, and may occur with smaller infarcts when there are additional neonatal factors.[65] Preterm infants with PAIS had more associated problems, such as language delay, than term infants.

Recurrence Risk

The recurrence risk for stroke appears to be very low. The Childhood Stroke Study Group followed up 215 neonates with arterial ischemic stroke for a median time of 3.5 years, during which time 7 children (3.3%) developed symptomatic thromboembolism (AIS, CSVT, or deep vein thrombosis of the leg). Four children developed a second AIS (~2%). Five children had a prothrombotic risk factor, and the second event was often triggered by a specific underlying problem such as infection, cardiac abnormality, or moyamoya disease.[13]

CEREBRAL SINOVENOUS THROMBOSIS
Incidence

The Canadian registry, one of the largest cohorts of pediatric stroke, estimated the incidence of cerebral venous thrombosis as at least 0.67 per 100,000 children per year,[66,67] whereas a German study estimated this at a higher rate of 2.6 per 100,000.[68] Neonates were the most frequently affected age group and accounted for 43% of cases in the Canadian registry. The estimated incidence of neonatal CSVT was 40.7 per 100,000 live births per year. This figure is likely to be an underestimate of the true incidence because the clinical presentation is nonspecific, the diagnosis may be missed clinically in the presence of coexistent illnesses occurring in the sick neonate, and the radiological diagnosis itself is not always straightforward, though it is easier to make in the acute phase. Not all CSVT is recognized to be symptomatic, and some CSVT clearly remains undiagnosed in neonatal or later life. In some cases the diagnosis is made on the basis of imaging performed for other reasons. A high index of suspicion is required to make the clinical and radiological diagnosis.

Pathophysiology and Risk Factors

CSVT has been associated with all the thrombotic risk factors that have been implicated in PAIS, such as Protein C or Protein S deficiency, G20210A prothrombin mutation, factor V Leiden mutation, antiphospholipid antibodies, infection, and polycythemia. Prothrombotic abnormalities have been reported in 15% to 20% of neonates with CSVT. A recent study comparing presumed PAIS and venous infarction in neonates found that there were no differences in prothrombotic conditions between the two groups.[69] However, children with presumed perinatal AIS were more likely to have acute perinatal risk factors (66% vs 17%, P = .002) including fetal distress, emergency cesarean section, or neonatal resuscitation. This finding is supported by a meta-analysis of 1764 patients in published observational studies, which reviewed the impact of thrombophilia on risk of first childhood stroke.[70] A statistically significant association with first stroke was demonstrated for each thrombophilia trait evaluated, with no difference found between AIS and CSVT. Venous sinus thrombosis and venous infarction may coexist with AIS in the same patient (Fig. 7).

In CVST there is often a history of an acute neonatal illness, for example an infection, meningitis, or dehydration, and other comorbidities such as neonatal congenital heart disease are common. Associated acute systemic illnesses at the time of diagnosis were present in the majority (61%–84%) of cases. Five percent of all infants with ECMO have evidence of CSVT. Complicated delivery is a common finding in CSVT, and traumatic delivery may disrupt the superior sagittal sinus or cortical veins. Maternal factors such as maternal diabetes and preeclampsia are also recognized.

The lesions detected in cerebral venous thrombosis are thrombus within an occluded or partially occluded vein or venous sinus, venous ischemia, venous infarction, and hemorrhage. Following

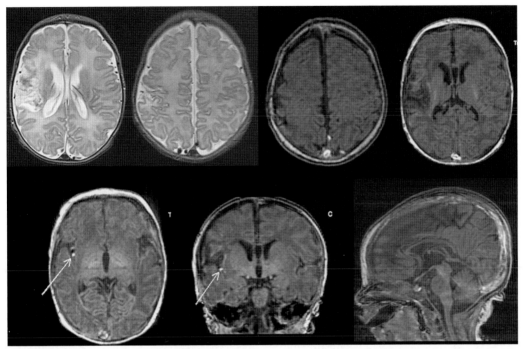

Fig. 7. MR imaging scans on a term baby born by cesarean section for failure to progress, scanned on day 14. The baby was born in good condition and no resuscitation was required. He went to the postnatal ward and breast fed well. At 36 hours of age, during a routine postnatal check he was noted to have left focal fits. His eyes fixed to the left and some nystagmus was noted. EEG showed right focal fits involving the left arm and ultrasonography showed a wedge-shaped area of increased echogenicity in the frontoparietal lobes. A maturing right MCA infarct is noted within the right frontoparietal lobes. The right MCA within the sylvian fissure is enlarged and shows signal abnormality, in keeping with thrombus (*arrows*). There is also evidence of extensive thrombus within the superior sagittal sinus that was not detected on the ultrasonography. The seizures resolved in the first week of life.

venous sinus thrombosis there is retrograde transmission of raised venous pressure proximal to the level of venous obstruction. This process increases both the venular and capillary hydrostatic pressure, which results in leakage of the capillary fluid into the interstitial space, causing vasogenic edema. The fluid leakage is often accompanied by red blood cells and is the usual cause of hemorrhagic venous infarcts in CSVT. Most of the edema is vasogenic and hence reversible but, if the process progresses, the capillary hydrostatic pressure and interstitial pressure can exceed the arteriolar pressure. This process can sometimes cause true venous infarction in which impairment of both arterial inflow and venous outflow occur.

Clinical Presentation

The diagnosis of CSVT should be considered in neonates presenting with seizures and encephalopathy, but the presentation may be more subtle and nonspecific and may include lethargy, apnea, and poor feeding, much like PAIS in this period. Around half of neonates present within the first 2 days of life and another 25% in the first week of life. Seizures may be subtle and focal or generalized. Some infants have relatively mild symptoms of encephalopathy despite extensive thrombosis within the venous sinuses. It is also recognized that venous sinus thrombosis may be detected as an incidental finding on brain MR imaging performed for other reasons.

Imaging

CSVT may be detected and missed on all imaging modalities, and in general isolated cortical vein thrombosis is not reliably and consistently diagnosed on any modality. However, because of the greater coverage achievable of the deep and superficial venous structures and superior evaluation of the brain parenchyma, CT and MR imaging are preferable to ultrasonography. MR imaging remains the modality of choice, as it does not involve ionizing radiation and is the most sensitive technique for detecting parenchymal lesions.

On unenhanced CT in the acute stage the involved venous sinuses appear hyperdense and expanded, the "dense triangle" or "cord sign" (**Fig. 8**). It can sometimes be difficult to discriminate

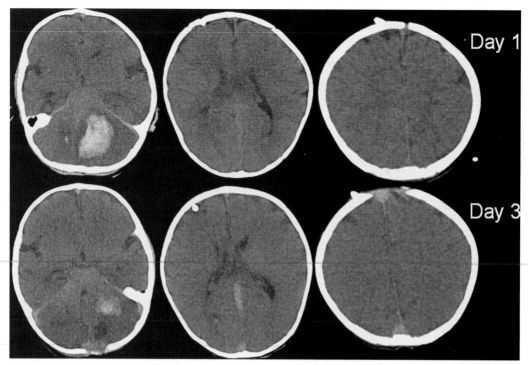

Fig. 8. CT scan (*top row*) in a 6-week-old infant with acute cerebellar hemorrhages causing marked cerebellar swelling presumed to be secondary to idiopathic thrombocytopenic purpura (no underlying structural lesion was found on follow-up MR imaging or angiography). A CT scan the day after the posterior fossa hematoma resection shows there is new acute thrombus in the straight sinus, torcular, and superior sagittal sinus.

between normal appearances of the neonatal venous sinuses, in which blood appears relatively hyperdense compared with the adjacent brain (**Fig. 9**). This normal appearance in the neonate is the result of a combination of persistent fetal hemoglobin and raised hematocrit; together they increase electron density in blood within the venous sinuses and hence increase the attenuation of x-rays. In addition, there is greater contrast between the relatively hyperdense normal neonatal venous sinus and the relatively low-density unmyelinated neonatal brain. The use of contrast, either a delayed postcontrast CT of the brain or a CT venogram, may facilitate the detection of nonenhancing thrombus, the "empty delta" or "empty triangle" sign.

On MR imaging a combination of T1-/T2-weighted sequences in multiple planes, as well as MR venography, are often necessary to make the diagnosis and avoid artifacts. Reliance on a single sequence, including MR venography, may lead to underdiagnosis or overdiagnosis (**Fig. 10**).[71] One observation and potential pitfall of 2-dimensional time-of-flight MR venography in neonates is that there seem to be more gaps in flow in the venous sinuses, particularly the posterior aspect of the superior sagittal sinus, which has been attributed to the age-related smaller size of the sinus, reduced venous flow, and skull molding.[72]

The brain itself may appear normal, or there may be diffuse cerebral swelling secondary to venous hypertension and ischemia. Lack of focal brain lesions or venous infarcts may not correlate with a good outcome (see **Fig. 10**). Enlargement of the ventricles can occur as a result of impaired venous outflow or be secondary to obstruction from associated intraventricular hemorrhage in deep venous infarction. Typically focal edematous brain parenchymal lesions involve the cortex and white matter, are seen in a typical venous tributary, and often have large intralesional hemorrhagic components early on or at presentation. There is some evidence that both brain lesions and hemorrhage are more common in neonates and infants than in children with CSVT.[73] It has been suggested that the mechanisms for compensation of raised intracranial pressure in neonates, such as opening up of reserve capillaries (increasing cerebral blood volume) or end-to-end meningeal anastomoses allowing alternative venous drainage, are immature in the neonate, making them more susceptible to venous ischemia and hemorrhage.

These edematous parenchymal lesions may have a mixed pattern of signal changes on diffusion-weighted imaging, with regions of increased and reduced diffusion on diffusion-weighted imaging/ADC maps. In the acute phase, imaging does not reliably

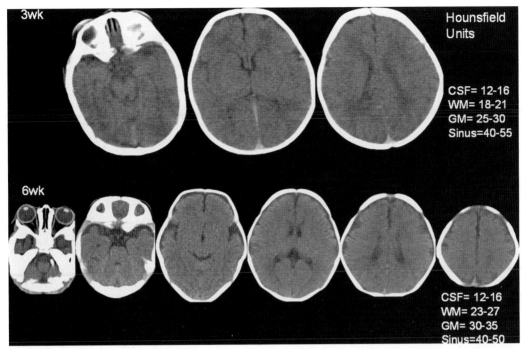

Fig. 9. Normal CT brain studies at 3 and 6 weeks of life. There is lower density within the white matter (WM) and gray matter (GM) on the earlier neonatal scan compared with the later one (visually and as measured in Hounsfield units). The venous sinuses appear relatively hyperdense in contrast to the lower-density brain. The sinus itself is also slightly more dense than on the later scan. However, there is no expansion of the sinus on any of the scans. CSF, cerebrospinal fluid. (*Courtesy of* WK "Kling" Chong, Great Ormond Street Hospital.)

discriminate between venous ischemia and venous infarction, even when diffusion-weighted imaging shows evidence of restricted diffusion. Unlike most AIS, these lesions have the potential to reverse with the development of alternative venous drainage pathways or recanalization of the venous sinus. Serial imaging should be considered if there is neurologic deterioration or hemorrhage in order to detect propagation of thrombus as well as progression of brain changes, as both may affect decisions to treat with anticoagulation. In a consecutive cohort study, asymptomatic thrombus propagation occurred in 25% of untreated neonatal CSVT compared with 3% of those who were treated with anticoagulation.[74] The AHA guideline also considers it reasonable to repeat imaging to assess for recanalization of the venous sinus in order to guide management.

Site

The venous drainage of the cerebral hemispheres is divided into the superficial and the deep systems. The superficial system consists of the superior sagittal sinus, the transverse sinuses, torcula, sigmoid sinuses, and the internal jugular veins. The deep system consists of the deep basal veins draining into the paired internal cerebral veins that unite with the inferior sagittal sinus and then drain into the vein of Galen, the straight sinus, and the torcula. Thrombus may propagate along the course of either system and may interconnect. As for the arterial tree in the neonate, the anatomic structure and distribution (though not necessarily the dynamic flow) of the major cerebral veins and venous sinuses are already established by the end of the first trimester. However, there is greater normal variation in the anatomic venous drainage and collateral venous drainage than in the arterial system, which leads to some variability in the distribution of parenchymal lesions in CSVT. Specific patterns of involvement include parasagittal subcortical hemorrhage with superior sagittal sinus thrombosis (the most common), thalamic and intraventricular hemorrhage with occlusion of the internal cerebral vein (**Fig. 11**), striatohippocampal hemorrhage with basal vein thrombosis, temporal lobe or cerebellar hemorrhage with transverse sinus thrombosis, temporal lobe anterolateral hemorrhage with tentorial sinus or temporal diploic vein rupture, and temporal lobe

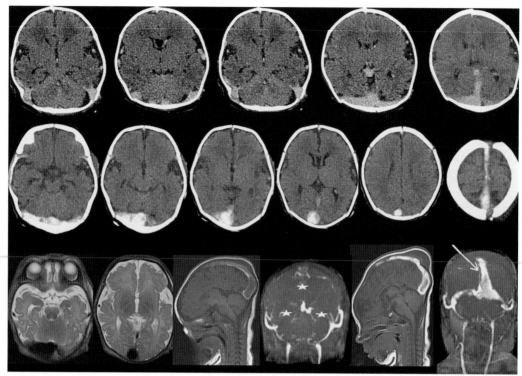

Fig. 10. A term male neonate who was unexpectedly hypotonic at birth with poor respiratory effort requiring resuscitation, and who developed seizures at 12 hours of life. His mother had reported unusual movements in utero. Initial CT (*top row*) on day 2 of life shows diffuse brain oedema, with expanded and hyperdense transverse and sagittal sinuses, torcula, and internal cerebral veins as well as the cerebral cortical veins. CT performed on day 9 (*middle row*) shows resolution of the cerebral oedema, increased density of the thrombus within the transverse sinus, torcula, and superior sagittal sinus. MR imaging on day 9 (*bottom left*, images 1–4) shows mild diffuse cerebral atrophy but no focal venous infarcts, with persistent thrombus and no flow on the MR venography (*stars*). Follow-up MR imaging on day 15 shows evolution of thrombus signal intensity to methemoglobin. Note the effect of T1 shortening within the thrombosed sagittal and transverse sinuses and torcula, mimicking flow within the sinuses (*arrow*). His seizures continued and were refractory to medical treatment. EEG continued to show interictal burst suppression pattern with multifocal epileptiform abnormalities. He subsequently died following uncontrolled seizures and respiratory arrest.

hemorrhage with vein of Labbe thrombosis. Deep venous anomalies may also thrombose in the presence of other risk factors (**Fig. 12**).

Treatment

The optimal treatment for neonatal SVT remains under debate. The mainstay of treatment is supportive with correction of dehydration, sepsis, anemia. Investigation of prothrombotic disorders and septic screening should be instituted. Kenet and colleagues[70] suggest anticoagulation should be given on an individual basis in children with newly identified SVT and high risk of recurrence. A recent Cochrane review in all patients with CSVT concluded that evidence was limited, but that anticoagulant treatment of cerebral venous sinus thrombosis appeared to be safe and was

associated with a potentially important reduction in the risk of death or dependency, although this did not reach statistical significance.[75] Treatment of neonatal CSVT with anticoagulation has not been universally accepted, and in the AHA guideline on pediatric stroke it was recognized that many neonates with CSVT are not treated, even in the presence of a thrombophilic disorder. The current AHA recommendation is that anticoagulation is a reasonable treatment option, even in the presence of hemorrhage, for 3 to 6 months. A clear distinction between symptomatic and asymptomatic infants is not made. Thrombolytic therapy with tissue plasminogen activator may be considered in selected children with CSVT (Class IIb, level of evidence C). The American College of Chest Physicians guideline (2008), however, concluded that, as for AIS, there are insufficient data to

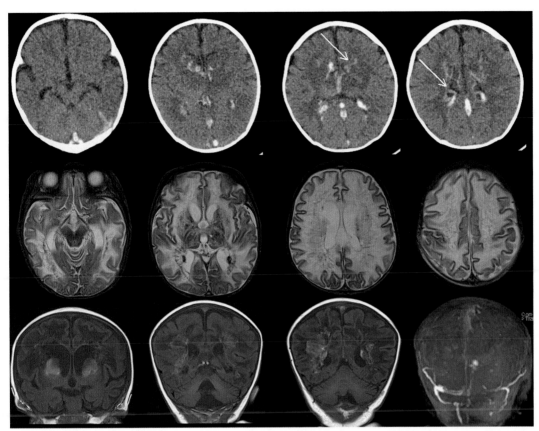

Fig. 11. On day 20 of life this baby girl was admitted to the pediatric intensive care unit with seizures and encephalopathy with hypernatremic dehydration, following rotavirus gastroenteritis. During her admission she also developed left femoral vein thrombosis extending into the inferior vena cava and superficial femoral artery thrombosis following insertion of vascular catheters, despite being treated with intravenous heparin. Her Protein S levels were found to be low after the acute illness and her mother also had low Protein S levels. CT of the brain shows hyperdensity in the internal cerebral veins, vein of Galen, straight, transverse, and occipital sinuses, as well as within ependymal and septal veins (*arrows*). She has low-density changes with swelling in the thalami and swelling and haemorrhage within the basal ganglia. Follow-up MR imaging 3 months later shows extensive infarction of the white matter, with linear signal abnormality suggestive of thrombosis or hemorrhage within or around the medullary veins. There is mature hemorrhagic infarction of the basal ganglia and thalami.

recommend more invasive treatment by thrombolysis (intravenous or intra-arterial) or thrombectomy outside a randomized controlled clinical trial.

Outcome

CSVT is associated with significant morbidity and mortality. Adverse outcomes include postnatal epilepsy, cerebral palsy, visual deficits, cognitive impairments, posthemorrhagic hydrocephalus requiring shunting, and death.[57,76,77] It is not clear how outcomes in neonates differ from those in children, although one study found higher mortality rates of CSVT in neonates.[78] A recent study showed that in 52 neonates with SVT, moderate to severe neurologic sequelae were present in 38% and 19% (10 infants) died. Normal neurodevelopment was seen in only 45%.[79] Neurologic deficits appear to be related to the presence of multiple venous sinus involvement and the presence of venous infarctions.

Recurrence

There are few data on the recurrence risk of CSVT in neonates. In the cohort of 396 children with CSVT studied by Kenet and colleagues,[80] none of the 22 children with recurrent thrombosis were younger than 2 years at the time of the initial thrombosis, implying that the risk of CSVT recurrence is low among very young children. However, children with more than one inherited thrombophilic factor who had venous thrombosis in the neonatal period may be at increased risk of future thrombotic events.[81] Additional data on the recurrence risk in different age groups are needed.

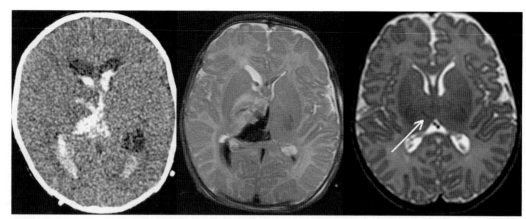

Fig. 12. A 1-month-old baby fasted for a research brain MR imaging performed 1 week previously in another unit. The baby had been unwell since the scans and had a more recent 24-hour history of fits and being floppy. CT and MR imaging of the brain (*left, middle*) show acute thrombus within a deep thalamic vein with thalamic edema, hemorrhage, and intraventricular hemorrhage. The scan prior to the acute illness shows the nonthrombosed deep venous anomaly (*arrow*).

GERMINAL MATRIX HEMORRHAGE-INTRAVENTRICULAR HEMORRHAGE AND PERIVENTRICULAR HEMORRHAGIC INFARCTION

Definition and Classification

Germinal matrix hemorrhage(GMH)-intraventricular hemorrhage (IVH) is bleeding that is confined to the germinal matrix or associated with uncomplicated intraventricular hemorrhage, with no evidence of ventricular enlargement. This terminology clearly separates GMH-IVH from parenchymal lesions. Periventricular hemorrhagic infarction refers to hemorrhagic necrosis of the periventricular white matter. This lesion frequently coexists with IVH; approximately 15% of all infants with GMH-IVH also exhibit periventricular hemorrhagic infarction. The traditional Papile classification graded hemorrhagic lesions in the preterm brain on a scale of I to IV on the basis of a single CT scan, and assumed parenchymal hemorrhage was simply the extension of blood from the ventricles.[82] This classification has been abandoned by some investigators because it does not allow for changes on serial imaging (improvement or progression) and assumes there is a continuous spectrum of abnormalities with hydrocephalus seen only with more severe lesions, and with grade IV parenchymal hemorrhage seen as the end stage of disease.[83]

Incidence

The incidence of GMH-IVH is inversely related to gestational age and birth weight. The incidence overall has been declining in Europe and the United States from around 50% in the 1970s to approximately 20% now,[84] due to improved care of preterm babies, unlike the incidence of periventricular leukomalacia. However, this overall reduction has not been seen in very low birth weight infants (<750 g), for whom periventricular hemorrhagic infarction (PVHI) is a particular problem.[85] It remains a bigger problem at all gestational ages outside Western countries; in one recent study from Syria the incidence of GMH-IVH was 44% of all neonates younger than 37 weeks.[86] GMH-IVH and PVHI mostly occur during early neonatal life, and 80% to 90% develop within the first 96 hours after birth with less than 20% being already present at birth. Only a minority (3%) have established lesions with porencephalic cysts on neonatal cranial ultrasound scans.

Pathophysiology and Risk Factors

The ganglionic eminence is thickest at 20 to 26 weeks gestational age and has involuted by 34 to 36 weeks.[87] Proliferative cells are numerous in both the ventral and dorsal ganglionic eminences until 18 weeks, after which there is a marked reduction in proliferative cells within the dorsal ganglionic eminence, while proliferative cells are still seen in the ventral ganglionic eminence until 28 weeks.

The developing neocortex is recognized to have several layers including the deep proliferative zones, which are clearly seen on postmortem MR imaging of the fetus. By 7 gestational weeks, the ventricular zone immediately surrounding the ventricular cavity gives rise to a secondary proliferative region, the subventricular zone (as well as the preplate, a precursor to the cortical layer). The intermediate zone, a precursor of the white matter, appears by 8 weeks. By 14 gestational weeks, the outer subplate and cortical plate have developed. Cortical projection neurons with long axons are generated from the ventricular zone mainly during the embryonic and early fetal period. The subventricular zone becomes the predominant site of cell generation after 15 weeks when it begins to expand rapidly in some sites, forming prominent ganglionic eminences along the lateral walls of the frontal horns, and to a lesser extent the temporal horns of the lateral ventricles. The ganglionic eminence (germinal matrix) is the source of neocortical γ-aminobutyric acid–ergic inhibitory interneurons, produced until at least 20 gestational weeks, and neurons for the adjacent basal ganglia, produced until 25 weeks. Neuron production for the thalamus, likely to be from the ventral ganglionic eminence, continues until 34 weeks. The subventricular zone also generates precursors of oligodendrocytes and astrocytes well into the third trimester. The germinal matrix then regresses gradually, with eventual involution of the ganglionic eminence by 34 to 36 gestational weeks.

GMH most often arises from the ganglionic eminence, which lies between the frontal horn of the lateral ventricle and the head of the caudate nucleus. The germinal matrix vasculature seems to be inherently vulnerable to reduced cerebral blood flow, due to factors such as discontinuous glial end feet of the blood-brain barrier, relative lack of pericytes, immature basal lamina, relatively thin vessel walls, and increased angiogenicity with increased endothelial turnover.[88]

In animal models there is evidence of direct toxicity of plasma, serum, thrombin, and plasmin on the perinatal subventricular zone in rats; these affect proliferation, differentiation, and migration in oligodendrocyte precursor cell cultures. In another animal experiment, unilateral injection of autologous blood into the periventricular region led to bilateral reduced cell proliferation in the germinal matrix from 8 hours to 1 week following injection, leading to increased cell death in the ipsilateral striatum by 2 days, with peak astrocytic and glial reaction seen at 2 days and persisting for up to 4 weeks. Three mechanisms are suggested for GMH: inherent fragility of the germinal matrix vasculature, disturbance in cerebral blood flow, then additional platelet and coagulation disorders that result in expansion (rather than initiation) of a spontaneous GMH.[89]

Again maternal, neonatal, and obstetric risk factors may all play a part. GMH-IVH is associated with vaginal delivery, low birth weight, low Apgar scores, hypoxia and hypercapnia, fetomaternal infection, and expression of inflammatory cytokines. Very low birth weight infants who are carriers for Factor V Leiden or prothrombin gain-of-function mutations are also at increased risk for development of GMH-IVH. Genetic factors act as independent risk factors of the same magnitude as other known risk factors.[90]

PVHI is thought to arise following bleeding into the germinal matrix, and not as extension of hemorrhage from IVH into the adjacent parenchyma.[91] Essentially this is a venous infarct. The medullary veins have a fanlike appearance within the frontal lobe white matter adjacent to the basal ganglia, and converge to a single draining terminal vein within the germinal matrix. GMH causes obstruction to the medullary venous outflow, and thrombus within the medullary veins may develop. Venous ischemia and eventually infarction with hemorrhagic necrosis may occur as a consequence of impaired venous outflow. The hemorrhagic component of the infarction tends to be most concentrated near the junction of the frontal horn with the body of the lateral ventricle. At this location the fan-shaped medullary veins draining the cerebral white matter converge, forming a sharp angle to join the terminal vein running along the wall of the lateral ventricle. PVHI is a pathologic entity distinct from periventricular leukomalacia, in which secondary hemorrhage may occur as the result of a reperfusion injury following watershed ischemic damage to the white matter in the preterm infant, and also from the white matter injury that may be seen with untreated hydrocephalus. Because neuroimaging may not always clearly delineate the underlying mechanism, some investigators prefer usage of the simpler term intraparenchymal lesion, which does not attribute any particular etiology to the lesion.

Imaging

Ultrasonography is usually the first neuroimaging study performed on the preterm brain. The main limitations of cranial ultrasonography are the subjectivity of interpretation and lack of interobserver correlation. Accurate interpretation depends on training and experience.[92] The detection of parenchymal lesions and intraventricular hemorrhage demonstrates greater agreement between observers than for GMH. Another study found that compared with MR imaging, ultrasonography accurately predicted the presence of GMH, IVH, and hemorrhagic parenchymal infarction on MR imaging.[93] However, intraobserver agreement is greater for MR imaging than for ultrasonography, and some studies have shown greater agreement than ultrasonography of postmortem findings.

GMH is typically seen on ultrasonography as an echogenic region in the caudothalamic groove, and must be distinguished from the mildly echogenic appearance of the normal choroid plexus, which may also be seen in the caudothalamic groove and is potentially a cause of misdiagnosis. Associated intraventricular hemorrhage may be seen as intraventricular echogenic areas extending from the caudothalamic groove, often forming dependent blood-cerebrospinal fluid levels or casts of hemorrhage around the choroid plexus within the lateral ventricles. Associated ventricular dilatation due to either hydrocephalus secondary to obstruction at the foramina of Monro/cerebral aqueduct or generalized white matter loss may be present.

MR imaging used for prognostic purposes is ideally performed in preterm infants at term gestational age. Imaging at this time allows comparisons with the published MR imaging literature for detection of abnormality versus the normal neonatal brain at term. On MR imaging the germinal matrix is most prominent in the second trimester fetus at 24 and 26 weeks of gestation, and forms a band of low intensity on T2-weighted MR images along the lateral margin of the lateral ventricles. GMH is seen typically as darker linear regions on T2-weighted sequences in the caudothalamic region or along the lateral ventricular ependyma, due to either deoxyhemoglobin or more usually hemosiderin. Acute hydrocephalus is most accurately distinguished from white matter volume loss by the presence of temporal horn distension and distension of the inferior and posterior recesses of the third ventricle. Unlike ultrasonography, MR imaging may clearly show the obstructive hemorrhagic lesion, for example as a focus of hemorrhage obstructing the cerebral aqueduct or foramina of Monro, and also may show intraventricular septations that may help to guide placement of ventricular drains and third ventriculostomy.

PVHI or parenchymal venous infarction is seen as a focal region, typically fan shaped, extending from the level of the caudothalamic groove into the adjacent brain. More than half of cases are asymmetric. The thrombosed veins may be demonstrated. On ultrasonography the PVHI is seen as a region of echogenicity in the basal ganglia and thalami with its apex at the caudothalamic groove, and on MR imaging as a region of signal change in keeping with either hemorrhage, edema, or a combination of the two. It is asymmetric in most cases. As the coagulation necrosis resolves there is tissue loss and a porencephalic cyst develops, which is usually, but not exclusively, in continuity with the lateral ventricle (**Fig. 13**). If the lesion has occurred in the early preterm period (<26 weeks gestational age) when the brain does not respond to insults with gliosis, then this cyst is typically smooth walled with no evidence of surrounding signal abnormality. Later than this there may be evidence of white matter scarring adjacent to the cyst (**Figs. 14** and **15**). The main differential diagnosis is from the cysts or white matter scars of focal periventricular leukomalacia; these are usually smaller, bilateral, and not so asymmetric, are seen more posteriorly within the white matter, and are more often associated with a worse outcome. Cerebellar hemorrhages are frequently seen in the presence of supratentorial GMH, PVHI, and white matter injury (**Fig. 16**)

PVHI is well described in infants delivered preterm but may occur in utero; it may also be detected prenatally or may present as presumed perinatal ischemic stroke in infancy following term birth. Familial porencephaly is an autosomal dominant condition in which leukoencephalopathy, macrohemorrhages and microhemorrhages, and porencephalic cysts occur, while adults may present with hemorrhages, small vessel disease, and intracranial aneurysms. It is a cause of strokes at any age,[94] may also affect infants and fetuses[95,96] and may mimic the appearances of PVHI. Recently a mutation in the gene encoding a protein of collagen type 4 A1 has been identified that impairs the structural integrity of the vascular basal membrane, rendering vessels susceptible to rupture. The porencephalic cysts are presumed to have occurred as a consequence of preterm hemorrhage and have an appearance similar to the mature injury seen following PVHI, but in the absence of a clinical history of preterm delivery or neonatal illness. An additional clue may be the presence of cataracts (**Fig. 17**).

Outcome

The traditional Papile ultrasound grading predicts morbidity and mortality, with ultrasonographic grades III (intraventricular hemorrhage with ventricular dilatation) and IV (intraventricular hemorrhage complicated by periventricular hemorrhagic infarction). Grade III hemorrhage has survival rates of 67% and 40%, respectively. Neurologic sequelae are seen in 50% of Grade III and 75% of Grade IV hemorrhages.

More than half of babies who have a porencephalic cyst will develop a contralateral hemiplegia in childhood. The majority of surviving preterm children with periventricular hemorrhagic infarction in one study had cerebral palsy with limited functional impairment at school age.[97] Infants with unilateral PVHI had better motor and cognitive outcomes than infants with bilateral PVHI.[98] This finding seems to be related to the anatomic site

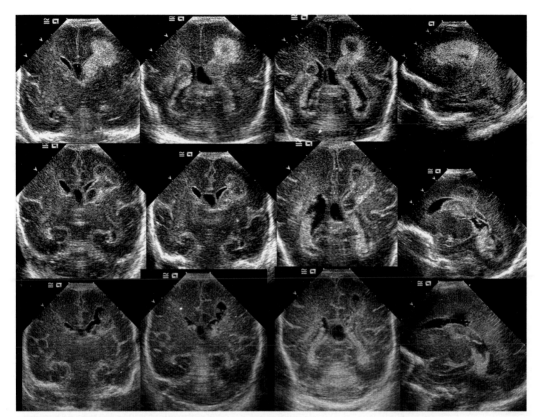

Fig. 13. Ultrasound images of one of twins born at 25 gestational weeks showing evolution of an acute left basal ganglia, intraventricular and frontal white matter hemorrhage into a region of porencephaly in continuity with the ventricle (*Top row* day 3, *middle row* day 16, *bottom row* day 54). (*Courtesy of* Cornelia Hagmann, Neonatal Unit, University College Hospital, London.)

of the cyst and whether it involves the CST. Hence anterior cysts have a better prognosis than posterior frontal or parietal cysts,[99,100] and MR imaging does have some advantages here in both accurately localizing the cyst and its relation to the corticospinal tract as well as in the detection of abnormal signal in the CST within the posterior limb of the internal capsule (see **Fig. 14**). This finding correlates with a higher incidence of contralateral hemiplegia in such infants compared with babies who have normal-appearing myelin within the CST. Abnormal signal may be seen remote from the cyst itself along the course of the CST, and is presumably caused by Wallerian degeneration. If there is coexistent ventricular enlargement due to white matter loss (eg, following untreated hydrocephalus or additional hypoxic-ischemic white matter injury), the risk of cognitive impairment is increased. Decreased cortical thickness has been found in uncomplicated GMH (without PVHI). GMH-IVH has an increased risk of major depressive disorder and obsessive-compulsive disorder by age 16 years.

INTRACEREBRAL HEMORRHAGE

Hemorrhagic stroke is less common than ischemic stroke in children,[101] and likely also less common in neonates, although the data on its incidence rate are lacking.[102] Much of the difficulty of estimating the prevalence of neonatal intracranial hemorrhage (ICH) in general is related to frequent occurrence of asymptomatic hemorrhages that may not come to clinical attention, and variable results attributable to different populations studied and sensitivity of diagnostic imaging tools.[102] Two reports estimated the regional incidence of symptomatic ICH in full-term infants at 4.9 and 5.9 per 10,000 live births, respectively.[103,104] However, another case-control study based on a northern California health maintenance practice from 1993 to 2003 estimated a lower prevalence for symptomatic perinatal hemorrhagic stroke (including intracerebral and subarachnoid hemorrhage) of 6.2 per 100,000 live births, about one-fifth the prevalence of symptomatic PAIS.[105] In recent years identification of ICH with intraparenchymal involvement has increased in neonates because of improved imaging techniques and increased

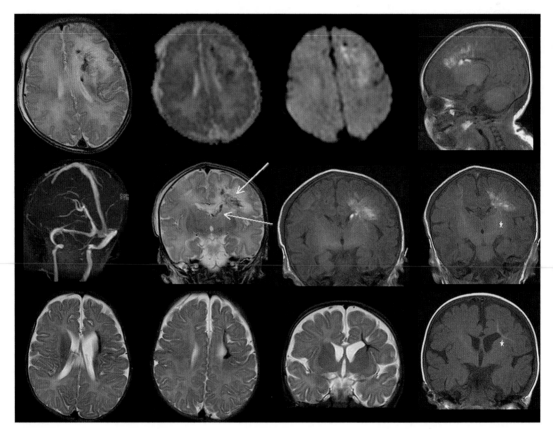

Fig. 14. MR images at day 3 of life (*top, middle rows*) in a male neonate born at 38 weeks gestational age following cesarean section for fetal distress and born with good Apgar scores of 8 and 9 at 1 and 5 minutes, respectively. On day 2 the baby developed seizures with sepsis, thrombocytopenia, hypoglycemia, polycythemia, jaundice, and respiratory distress syndrome. Initial ultrasound scans were reported as showing grade 2 intraventricular hemorrhage and a left frontal parenchymal lesion. The MR imaging shows left frontal lobe white matter edema with multiple linear regions consistent with thrombus in medullary veins, adjacent. The diffusion-weighted imaging shows areas of both increased diffusion and restriction or hemorrhage. Focal enlargement and signal change indicating methemoglobin is seen within ependymal and transverse caudate veins, and there is a typical fan-shaped appearance of the thrombosed medullary veins and surrounding edema on the coronal sections (*arrows*). The venous sinuses are patent. On follow-up MR imaging at 3 months (*bottom row*), there is small region of left frontal porencephaly with evidence of hemosiderin along its lateral margin as well as left frontal lobe atrophy. Note the asymmetrical myelination of the motor tract within the posterior limb of the internal capsule (*stars*). At assessment at 3 months of age, he had marginally increased tone in the right upper limb and the right fist was not as freely open as the left.

use of diagnostic imaging.[106] In this discussion, neonatal hemorrhagic stroke is mainly defined as acute stroke with intraparenchymal hemorrhage in infants during the first month of life.

Clinical Presentation

The most frequent presenting symptoms in both preterm and term newborns with ICH are neonatal seizure and decreased level of consciousness.[102] Depending on the site of hemorrhage, there may be cranial nerve palsy, hemiparesis, and apnea. Frequently there are also nonspecific signs such as lethargy, irritability, fever, cyanosis, crying, vomiting, or diarrhea. In a retrospective analysis

of 33 symptomatic term infants with ICH,[103] 24 of 33 infants (73%) presented with seizure, respiratory distress, or apnea. A subset of 4 patients who had lobar hemorrhage all manifested with seizures.[103,107] In another neuroimaging series of 53 term infants who had ICH with parenchymal involvement, seizures were found to be the most common presenting symptom (71.7%), and another 18.9% presented with apneic seizures while 5 infants (9.4%) had no clinical signs.[106]

Risk Factors

In children, a few risk factors for cerebral hemorrhage have been identified, including underlying

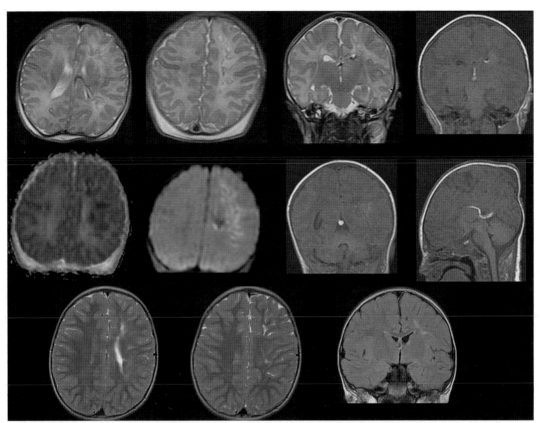

Fig. 15. MR brain scans (*top* and *middle* rows) in a term baby who had difficulty feeding after delivery, developed weight loss, and presented with apneic episodes. He was found to have hypernatremic dehydration, then developed left femoral vein thrombosis after vascular catheter insertion. EEG showed bilateral focal changes. Low Protein S level was found and confirmed 3 months later. There is thrombus within the left ependymal vein extending into the internal cerebral vein and vein of Galen. There is maturing left frontal lobe white matter infarction with linear signal abnormality, suggestive of thrombosis in the medullary veins. Follow-up imaging 2 years (*bottom row*) later shows mature white matter scarring, extending from the periventricular into the left frontal subcortical white matter with focal volume loss. This appearance could incorrectly be interpreted as periventricular leukomalacia, but the latter is usually bilateral, though it may be asymmetrical.

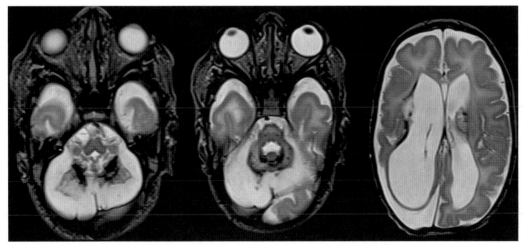

Fig. 16. MR images of a preterm infant scanned at term showing extensive cerebellar atrophy and mature cerebellar hemorrhages as well as bilateral germinal matrix hemorrhages. A focal region of porencephaly is seen on the right associated with greater enlargement of the right lateral ventricle.

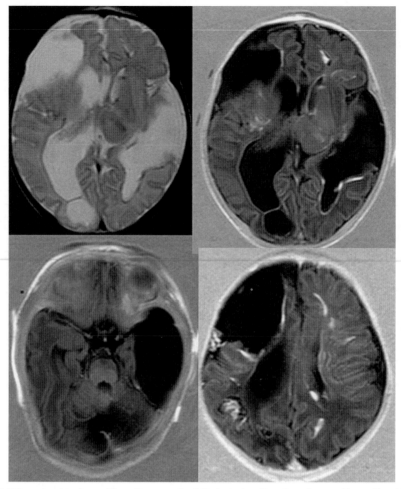

Fig. 17. Brain MR imaging in a boy with epilepsy and a 4-limb motor disorder who was 7 months at the time of his scan, showing multiple bilateral asymmetrical porencephalic cysts with scattered mature white matter hemorrhages. He has left microphthalmia and a congenital cataract, and a confirmed de novo mutation in the ColIVA1 gene.

coagulopathy, vascular malformation, malignancy, and trauma. A large population-based study of childhood stroke over a 10-year period from the 1970s identified 45% (31 of 69 all stroke cases) of hemorrhagic stroke comprising both subarachnoid and intracerebral hemorrhage.[108] The study included infants and children ranging in age from 0 to 14 years, and arteriovenous malformation (AVM) was cited as the most common cause of hemorrhagic stroke in children (18.8%) when stroke related to birth, intracranial infection, or trauma was excluded. Other vascular malformations that carried the risk of hemorrhage included cavernous malformation and aneurysm, the latter contributing to 8.7% of all hemorrhagic strokes in the same study.[108] Hemorrhage and venous ischemia may be seen in vein of Galen aneurysmal malformations (**Fig. 18**).

In neonates, the primary risk factors for hemorrhagic stroke include prematurity, underlying coagulopathic disorders (whether genetically predisposed or iatrogenically induced), trauma, and also underlying vascular malformations or malignancies. Of note, in a case-control study[105] using multivariant analysis, fetal distress and postmaturity were found to be the strongest independent predictors of perinatal hemorrhagic stroke. ICH and, in particular, intraventricular hemorrhage are most commonly seen in preterm newborns with low birth weight (<1500 g), most likely related to immature vasculature. In term newborns, on the other hand, intracranial hemorrhage is considered uncommon and often has a different, nonintraventricular (more frequently subdural, subarachnoid followed by intraparenchymal) location, etiology, and clinical presentation, as well as more variable

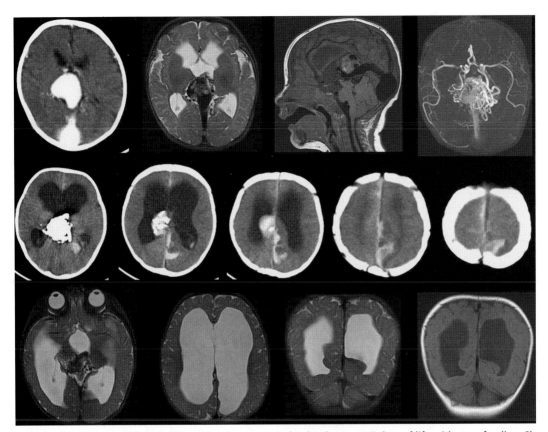

Fig. 18. A female neonate born at 38 weeks who was noted to be drowsy at 5 days of life with poor feeding. She had mild signs of cardiac failure. Chest radiography showed cardiomegaly, and cranial ultrasonography was reported to show an intracranial vascular malformation. CT scan (*top left*) confirmed vein of Galen aneurysmal malformation, which was partly treated by transarterial glue embolization without complication but with significant residual arteriovenous shunting (MR images *top row*). Following a second embolization procedure there was acute clinical deterioration with signs of raised intracranial pressure (hypertension, bradycardia, and reduced level of consciousness). CT of the brain showed acute intraventricular hemorrhage (IVH) and hydrocephalus, and a left parieto-occipital lobe low-density lesion with adjacent subarachnoid and subdural hematoma. Some linear hyperdensity was believed to be due to thrombus within the persistent falcine sinus. Follow-up imaging shows maturation of the focal left parieto-occipital lesion in keeping with an infarct, which is probably venous in origin.

neurologic outcome.[98] In the perinatal period, GMH is most frequently encountered in premature infants and is fully discussed in the previous section. The most advanced GMH, classified as Grade IV hemorrhage, includes a parenchymal component in addition to intraventricular hemorrhage. This periventricular hemorrhagic pattern may also be seen in term neonates, and was found in 9 of 33 (27.3%) term infants in the series of Hanigan and colleagues.[107]

Coagulopathy is a major risk factor for intracranial hemorrhage in both preterm and term neonates. A diagnosis of underlying coagulopathic disorder (whether due to production defects or functional abnormalities) should always be considered in neonates presenting with ICH.

Coagulopathies tend to make intracranial hemorrhage much more severe and devastating. Failure to give Vitamin K at birth is a recognised cause. Hemophilia A (due to deficiency of factor VIII) and hemophilia B (due to factor IX deficiency) are the most common severe inherited coagulopathies, and can both cause ICH. Hemophilia C, due to deficiency of factor XI, is much less common. Von Willebrand disease is rarely a cause of neonatal cerebral hemorrhage because the factor typically follows a physiologic elevation at birth, providing protection from bleeding.

Some of the genetic causes of coagulopathic disorders include glutaric aciduria type 1, a metabolic disorder that presents with retinal and intracranial (most often subdural) hemorrhages that are not nonaccidental. Congenital disorders of glycosylation is a spectrum of disorders that affects multiple organ systems with increased susceptibility to bleed, and several rare inborn errors of metabolism such as galactosemia (which can present with progressive lethargy, irritability, poor feeding, and liver dysfunction), tyrosinemia type I (worsening liver function with elevated transaminases, lethargy, and poor feeding that can progress to coagulopathy, distress, coma, and death), and carnitine/acylcarnitine translocase deficiency (liver failure and resultant hyperammonemia). Carnitine palmitoyltransferase 2 deficiency (CPT2 deficiency) has a severe neonatal form whereby there is evidence of liver failure with hypoglycemia, cardiomyopathy, and arrhythmias that presents within days of birth and can lead to seizures, and focal malformations of specific organs.

Much more frequently coagulation problems are acquired, and hemorrhagic stroke occurs because of sepsis or iatrogenic factors, for example, the use of anticoagulation in ECMO. Thrombocytopenia is the most common condition causing ICH in term newborns,[106,109] and has many causes including drug-induced, infectious, genetic, immune-mediated, disseminated intravascular coagulation, or placental insufficiency.[110] In the Kaiser pediatric stroke study based in northern California, thrombocytopenia accounted for 20% of perinatal hemorrhagic stroke while 75% were deemed idiopathic.[105]

Associated Pathophysiology

Based on previously published studies and the authors' own experience in examining intraparenchymal hemorrhage in term newborns, the underlying etiological factors remain unknown in many, sometimes up to 50%, of cases.[102–114,111] It is noteworthy that none of the cases in several reported studies involved an underlying arteriovenous malformation or neoplasm, while cavernous malformation accounted for 1 in 20 cases of the Kaiser study in a 10-year span.[105] The absence of AVM was documented in the series by Bergman and colleagues[111] by negative contrast CT scan and/or cerebral angiograms at the time of acute symptoms or on follow-up, and appears to be the common experience shared by other investigators.[103,106,107] Hence it seems that AVM, while a relatively common cause of hemorrhage in children, should not be generally be considered a cause of ICH in the neonate.

HIE and hemorrhagic injuries often occur concomitantly in both preterm and term newborns, and share many similar pathophysiologic and clinical features.[101] In the Bergman series[111] it was thought that most cases of intraparenchymal hemorrhage resulted from hemorrhagic infarction. In their retrospective review of patients under 1 month old with ICH within a span of 10 years since 1975, 18 term neonatal infants were identified, among whom 6 presented with primarily intraparenchymal hemorrhage. Two patients sustained hypoxic-ischemic injury, while one had hyperviscosity of blood predisposing to infarction. Three of these 6 patients did not have any identifiable precipitating conditions, but were postulated to have suffered from embolic hemorrhagic infarctions based on the distribution of haemorrhage and subsequent areas of cerebral damage seen on follow up CT. However hemorrhagic transformation of AIS can usually be excluded on MRI. Some lobar hemorrhages may be seen in association with thrombosed medullary veins or cortical veins (such as vein of L'Abbe in temporal lobe hematomas). However often the underlying cause is not identified.

Imaging

Neuroimaging is important in the evaluation of these neonates, and allows prompt and accurate diagnosis. Cranial ultrasonography is most frequently used as the first line of imaging modality, and has distinct advantages of portability, low cost, lack of ionizing radiation, and ease of operation for serial examinations. Ultrasonography is particularly useful in following preterm neonates, who are prone to GMH, and in infants treated with ECMO, without removing them from the intensive care unit or requiring sedation to be used. Hemorrhage is depicted on ultrasonography as increased echogenicity (**Fig. 19**), but the low contrast against the choroid plexus and adjacent brain tissue makes it difficult to resolve the small amount of hemorrhage and diffuse parenchymal abnormalities. CT and MR imaging are more sensitive in the detection of ICH than ultrasonography, and have superior capability of delineating blood in different compartments in addition to depicting other parenchymal abnormalities, such as those resulting from ischemia, with much greater interobserver agreement.[112–114] **Fig. 20** illustrates the conspicuous wedge-shaped hypoattenuation on CT representing arterial infarct, which subsequently undergoes hemorrhagic transformation with curvilinear hyperattenuation. MR imaging is even superior to CT in evaluating brain parenchyma particularly for concomitant ischemic changes, which have been found to be an important predictor of neurodevelopmental outcomes. Susceptibility-weighted imaging can highlight petechial hemorrhage that may offer clues to underlying pathophysiology (**Fig. 21**). In the same MR examination, MR angiography and MR

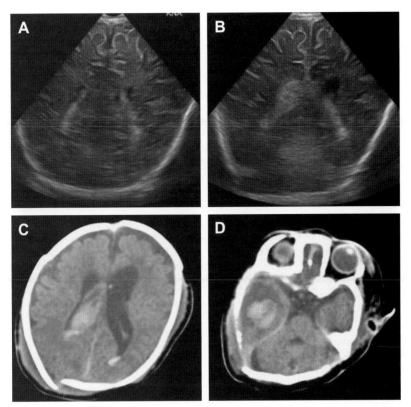

Fig. 19. A male infant born at 38 weeks with congenital diaphragmatic defect and pulmonary hypoplasia, treated with extracorporeal membrane oxygenation. (*A*) Baseline head ultrasonography is normal. (*B*) On day 15, ultrasonography shows increased echogenicity within the choroid plexus in the right lateral ventricle with ventricular dilation, suggesting IVH. (*C*) Noncontrast head CT performed on day 20 confirms hemorrhage casting the right lateral ventricle, in addition to a small amount of IVH in the left occipital horn, as well as moderate ventricular dilation. (*D*) Head CT also shows a new right temporal hematoma with surrounding vasogenic edema.

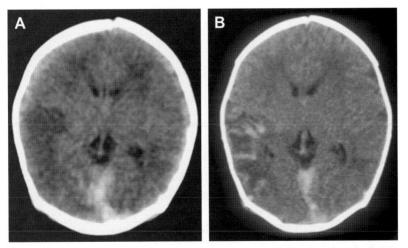

Fig. 20. A newborn baby boy with normal delivery and Apgar scores of 8 (1 minute) and 9 (5 minutes) presented with jerky movements of clonic nature suggestive of seizure at 2 hours of life. (*A*) Head CT shows a wedge-shaped hypoattenuation in the right parietal lobe consistent with right MCA territory infarct. (*B*) On day 10 of life, curvilinear densities are identified within the area of infarct, reflecting hemorrhagic conversion.

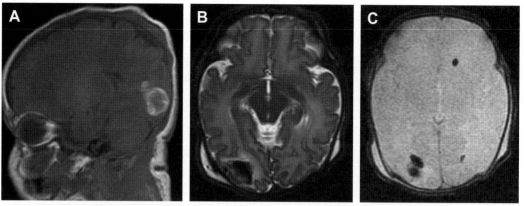

Fig. 21. A 35-week preterm baby boy born by cesarean section who had an uncomplicated delivery but developed pulmonary hypertension of newborn, resulting in hypoxic damage of his liver and kidney, and subsequently disseminated intravascular coagulation and intracranial hemorrhage. (*A*) T1-weighted sagittal MR image shows a peripherally hyperintense and centrally isointense hematoma in the occipital lobe. (*B*) T2-weighted axial image shows the right occipital hematoma is dark, reflecting acute hemorrhage with deoxyhemoglobin blood products and peripheral rim of intracellular methemoglobin. (*C*) T2*-weighted axial image shows several foci of parenchymal hemorrhage, possibly mixed with intraventricular blood.

venography can also easily be incorporated to allow interrogation of vascular abnormalities.

The hemoglobin products evolve with time through several forms including oxyhemoglobin, deoxyhemoglobin, and intracellular and extracellular methemoglobin, and finally get broken down to ferritin and hemosiderin, which are sequestered by macrophages and scavenger cells in the chronic stage. T1 shortening occurs in methemoglobin as a result of paramagnetic dipole-dipole interactions, whereas the magnetic susceptibility effect accounts for T2 shortening observed with deoxyhemoglobin, methemoglobin, and hemosiderin (see **Fig. 21**).[115] Five stages of hemorrhage are described on conventional MR imaging:

1. Hyperacute (intracellular oxyhemoglobin, long T1, long T2)
2. Acute (intracellular deoxyhemoglobin, long T1, short T2)
3. Early subacute (intracellular methemoglobin, short T1, short T2)
4. Late subacute (extracellular methemoglobin, short T1, long T2)
5. Chronic (ferritin and hemosiderin, short T2).

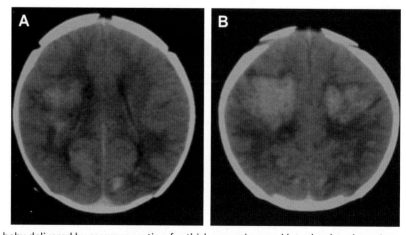

Fig. 22. Term baby delivered by cesarean section for thick meconium and late decelerations, Apgar scores of 1, 6, and 8 (at 1, 5, and 10 minutes), presented with neonatal seizures at night of first day of life. EEG showed bilateral hemispheric origin, all cultures were negative, and there was no evidence of venous sinus thrombosis. (*A, B*) Axial head CT images show bilateral frontal, parietal, and scattered occipital hemorrhages in the periventricular and subcortical white matter, the largest in the frontal centrum semiovale.

The pattern and location of hemorrhage may also offer some clues to the underlying etiology. For example, by examining the hematoma location and clinical factors in 25 term infants with ICH, Hanigan and colleagues[103] found periventricular hemorrhage (28% of all cases) (**Fig. 22**) and peripheral cortical hemorrhage (24%) predominantly associated with hypoxic-ischemic injury or coagulopathy. By contrast, lobar hemorrhage (16%) (**Fig. 23**) and extra-axial hemorrhage (32%) were often associated with trauma or coagulopathy. It would be of interest to confirm this association in a larger cohort of patients.

Outcomes

HIE has been cited as a major contributor to or associated clinical factor of intracranial hemorrhage.[103,111] Perinatal asphyxia and findings of cerebral ischemia are associated with a high mortality rate and poor neurodevelopmental outcomes.[103,106] The majority of infants with parenchymal hemorrhage from unknown causes had good Apgar scores. Long-term clinical outcome was found to be variable: 50% of those infants who suffered ICH had a normal development and 50% had moderate to severe disability.[111] The lobar type of hemorrhage described in the small series by Hanigan and colleagues[107] showed normal development in 3 out of 4 infants, but severe mental retardation in 1.

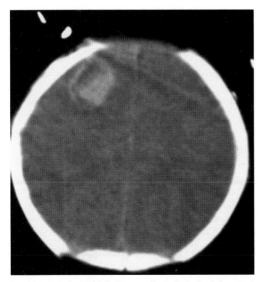

Fig. 23. A 1-day-old full-term female infant born via normal spontaneous vaginal delivery with forceps assistance, who was found to have a right frontal lobe hematoma following seizure activity at 15 hours of life. Axial head CT shows a hyperdense hematoma in the right frontal lobe.

REFERENCES

1. Ganesan V. Pediatric stroke guidelines: where will these take future research and treatment options for childhood stroke. Expert Rev Neurother 2009; 9(5):639–48.
2. Raju TN, Nelson KB, Ferriero D, et al. Ischemic perinatal stroke: summary of a workshop sponsored by the national institute of child health and human development and the national institute of neurological disorders and stroke. Pediatrics 2007;120:609–16.
3. Hall P, Adami HO, Trichopoulos D, et al. Effect of low doses of ionising radiation in infancy on cognitive function in adulthood: Swedish population based cohort study. BMJ 2004;328(7430):19.
4. Brenner DJ. Estimating cancer risks from pediatric CT: going from the qualitative to the quantitative. Pediatr Radiol 2002;32(4):228–31.
5. Estan J, Hope P. Unilateral neonatal cerebral infarction in full term infants. Arch Dis Child Fetal Neonatal Ed 1997;76:F88–93.
6. Schulzke S, Weber P, Luetschg J, et al. Incidence and diagnosis of unilateral arterial cerebral infarction in newborn infants. J Perinat Med 2005;33: 170–5.
7. Lee J, Croen LA, Backstrand KH, et al. Maternal and infant characteristics associated with perinatal arterial stroke in the infant. JAMA 2005;293(6):723–9.
8. Laugesaar R, Kolk A, Tomberg T, et al. Acutely and retrospectively diagnosed perinatal stroke: a population-based study. Stroke 2007;38:2234–40.
9. Benders MJ, Groenendaal F, De Vries LS. Preterm arterial ischemic stroke. Semin Fetal Neonatal Med 2009;14(5):272–7.
10. Nelson KB, Lynch JK. Stroke in newborn infants [review]. Lancet Neurol 2004;3:150–8.
11. Bushnell CD. Stroke in women: risk and prevention throughout the lifespan [review]. Neurol Clin 2008; 26(4):1161–76, xi.
12. Govaert P. Sonographic stroke templates. Semin Fetal Neonatal Med 2009;14(5):284–98.
13. Kurnik K, Kosch A, Strater R, et al. Recurrent thromboembolism in infants and children suffering from symptomatic neonatal arterial stroke. A prospective follow-up study. Stroke 2003;34: 2887–93.
14. Amelie-Lefond C, Bernard TJ, Sébire G, et al. International Pediatric Stroke Study Group. Predictors of cerebral arteriopathy in children with arterial ischaemic stroke: results of the International Pediatric Stroke Study. Circulation 2009;119(10):1417–23.
15. Roach ES. Etiology of stroke in children. Semin Pediatr Neurol 2000;7(4):244–60.
16. Sébire G, Fullerton H, Riou E, et al. Toward the definition of cerebral arteriopathies in childhood. Curr Opin Pediatr 2004;16(6):617–22.

17. Mackay MT, Wiznitzer M, Benedict SL, et al. International Pediatric Stroke Study Group. Arterial ischemic stroke risk factors: the international pediatric stroke study. Ann Neurol 2011;69(1):130–40.

18. Lequin MH, Peeters EA, Holscher HC, et al. Arterial infarction caused by carotid artery dissection in the neonate. Eur J Pediatr Neurol 2004;8:155–60.

19. Ganesan V, Cox TC, Gunny R. Abnormalities of cervical arteries in children with arterial ischemic stroke. Neurology 2011;76(2):166–71.

20. Chabrier S, Husson B, Dinomais M, et al. New insights (and new interrogations) in perinatal arterial ischemic stroke. Thromb Res 2011;127:13–22.

21. Gunther G, Junker R, Strater R, et al. Childhood stroke study group. Symptomatic ischemic stroke in full-term neonates: role of acquired and genetic prothrombotic risk factors. Stroke 2000;31:2437–41.

22. Benders MJ, Groenendaal F, Uiterwaal CS, et al. Maternal and infant characteristics associated with perinatal arterial stroke in the preterm infant. Stroke 2007;38:1759–65.

23. Golomb MR, Williams LS, Garg BP. Perinatal stroke in twins without co-twin demise. Pediatr Neurol 2006;35:75–7.

24. Mahle WT, Tavani F, Zimmerman RA, et al. An MRI study of neurological injury before and after congenital heart surgery. Circulation 2002;106 (12 Suppl 1):I109–14.

25. McQuillen PS, Barkovich AJ, Hamrick SE, et al. Temporal and anatomic risk profile of brain injury with neonatal repair of cardiac defects. Stroke 2007;38(Suppl 2):736–41.

26. Block AJ, McQuillen PS, Chau V, et al. Clinically silent preoperative brain injuries do not worsen with surgery in neonates with congenital heart disease. J Thorac Cardiovasc Surg 2010;140(3):550–7.

27. Chen J, Zimmerman RA, Jarvik GP, et al. Perioperative stroke in infants undergoing open heart operations for congenital heart disease. Ann Thorac Surg 2009;88(3):823–9.

28. Limperopoulos C, Tworetzy W, McElhinney DB. Brain volume and metabolism in fetuses with congenital heart disease. Circulation 2010;121:26–33.

29. Wernovsky G. Current insights regarding neurological and developmental abnormalities in children and young adults with complex congenital heart disease. Cardiol Young 2006;16(Suppl):92–104.

30. Ramaswamy V, Miller SP, Barkovich AJ, et al. Perinatal stroke in term infants with neonatal encephalopathy. Neurology 2004;62:2088–91.

31. Rennie J, Hagmann CF, Robertson NJ. The baby with suspected seizures. In: Neonatal cerebral investigation. Cambridge University Press; 2008. p. 103.

32. Elbers J, Viero S, MacGregor D, et al. Placental pathology in neonatal stroke. Pediatrics 2011; 127(3):e722–9.

33. Cheong JL, Cowan FM. Neonatal arterial ischemic stroke: obstetric issues. Semin Fetal Neonatal Med 2009;14:267–71.

34. Levy SR, Abroms IF, Marshall PC, et al. Seizures and cerebral infarction in the full-term newborn. Ann Neurol 1985;17(4):366–70.

35. Mercuri E, Barnett A, Rutherford M, et al. Neonatal cerebral infarction and neuromotor outcome at school age. Pediatrics 2004;113:95–100.

36. Kirton A, deVeber G. Cerebral palsy secondary to perinatal ischemic stroke. Clin Perinatol 2006;33: 367–86.

37. Wulfeck BB, Trauner DA, Tallal PA. Neurological, cognitive, and linguistic features of infants after early stroke. Pediatr Neurol 1991;7:266–9.

38. Mercuri E, Rutherford M, Cowan F, et al. Early prognostic indicators of outcome in infants with neonatal cerebral infarction: a clinical, electroencephalogram, and magnetic resonance imaging study. Pediatrics 1999;103:39–46.

39. Sreenan C, Bhargava R, Robertson CM. Cerebral infarction in the term newborn: clinical presentation and long-term outcome. J Pediatr 2000;137: 351–5.

40. Govaert P, Ramenghi L, Taal R, et al. Diagnosis of perinatal stroke 1: definitions, differential diagnosis and registration. Acta Paediatr 2009;98:1556–67.

41. De Vries LS, Groenendaal F, Eken P, et al. Infarcts in the vascular distribution of the middle cerebral artery in preterm and fullterm infants. Neuropediatrics 1997;28:88–96.

42. Perinatal disorders. In: Graham D, Lantos P, editors. Greenfield's neuropathology, vol. 1. 6th edition. London: Arnold; 1996.

43. Neumann-Haefelin T, Kastrup A, de Crespigny A, et al. Serial MRI after transient focal cerebral ischemia in rats: dynamics of tissue injury, blood-brain barrier damage and edema formation. Stroke 2000;31:1965–72.

44. Kuker W, Mohrle S, Mader I, et al. MRI for the management of neonatal cerebral infarctions: importance of timing. Childs Nerv Syst 2004;20: 742–8.

45. Dudink J, Mercuri E, Al-Nakib L, et al. Evolution of unilateral perinatal arterial ischemic stroke on conventional and diffusion-weighted MR imaging. AJNR Am J Neuroradiol 2009;30:998–1004.

46. Mader I, Schöning M, Klose U, et al. Neonatal cerebral infarction diagnosed by diffusion-weighted MRI: pseudonormalization occurs early. Stroke 2002;33:1142–5.

47. Fiebach JB, Jansen O, Schellinger PD, et al. Serial analysis of the apparent diffusion (ADC) abnormality in human stroke. Neuroradiology 2002;44: 294–8.

48. Lansberg MG, O'Brien MW, Tong DC, et al. Evolution of apparent diffusion coefficient, and

T2-weighted signal intensity of acute stroke. AJNR Am J Neuroradiol 2001;22:637–44.

49. Munoz Maniega A, Bastin ME, Armitage PA. Temporal evolution of water diffusion parameters is different in grey and white matter in human ischemic stroke. J Neurol Neurosurg Psychiatry 2004;75:1714–8.

50. Coker SB, Beltran RS, Myers TF, et al. Neonatal stroke: description of patients and investigation into pathogenesis. Pediatr Neurol 1988;4(4):219–23.

51. Perlman JM, Rollins NK, Evans D. Neonatal stroke: clinical characteristics and cerebral blood flow velocity measurements. Pediatr Neurol 1994;11(4):281–4.

52. Cowan F, Mercuri E, Groenendaal F, et al. Does cranial ultrasound imaging identify arterial cerebral infarction in term neonates? Arch Dis Child Fetal Neonatal Ed 2005;90:F252–6.

53. Boyko OB, Burger PC, Shelburne JD, et al. Non-heme mechanisms for T1 shortening: pathologic, CT, and MR elucidation. AJNR Am J Neuroradiol 1992;13(5):1439–45.

54. Fujikoya M, Taoka T, Matsuo Y, et al. Novel brain ischemic change on MRI. Delayed ischemic hyper-intensity on T1-weighted images and selective neuronal death in the caudoputamen of rats after brief focal ischemia. Stroke 1999;30:1043–6.

55. Niwa T, Aida N, Shishikura A, et al. Susceptibility-weighted imaging findings of cortical laminar necrosis in pediatric patients. AJNR Am J Neurora-diol 2008;29:1795–8.

56. De Veber G, Ferriero D, Jones BV, et al. Manage-ment of stroke in infants and children: a scientific statement from a special writing group of the Amer-ican Heart Association Stroke Council and the Council on Cardiovascular Disease in the Young. Stroke 2008;39:2644–91.

57. de Veber GA, MacGregor D, Curtis R, et al. Neuro-logical outcome in survivors of childhood arterial ischemic stroke and sinovenous thrombosis. J Child Neurol 2000;15(5):316–24.

58. Lynch JK, Nelson KB. Epidemiology of perinatal stroke. Curr Opin Pediatr 2001;13:499–505.

59. Walther M, Juenger H, Kuhnke N, et al. Motor cortex plasticity in ischemic perinatal stroke: a transcranial magnetic stimulation and functional MRI study. Pediatr Neurol 2009;41(3):171–8.

60. Boardman JP, Ganesan V, Rutherford MA, et al. Magnetic resonance imaging correlates of hemipa-resis after neonatal and childhood middle cerebral artery stroke. Pediatrics 2005;115(2):321–6.

61. Kirton A, Shroff M, Visvanathan T, et al. Quantified corticospinal tract diffusion restriction predicts neonatal stroke outcome. Stroke 2007;38:974–80.

62. Husson B, Hertz-Pannier L, Renaud C, et al. AVCnn Group. Motor outcomes after neonatal arterial ischemic stroke related to early MRI data in a prospective study. Pediatrics 2010;126(4):912–8.

63. Hunt RW, Inder TE. Perinatal and neonatal ischemic stroke: a review. Thromb Res 2006; 118(1):39–48.

64. Westmacott R, Askalan R, MacGregor D, et al. Cognitive outcome following unilateral arterial is-chaemic stroke in childhood: effects of age at stroke and lesion location. Dev Med Child Neurol 2010;5(2):386–93.

65. Ricci D, Mercuri E, Barnett A, et al. Cognitive outcome at early school age in term-born children with perinatally acquired middle cerebral artery territory infarction. Stroke 2008;3(9):403–10.

66. Schmidt B, Andrew M. Neonatal thrombosis: report of a prospective Canadian and international registry. Pediatrics 1995;96(5):939–43.

67. deVeber G, Andrew M, Adams C, et al. Childhood pediatric Ischemic Stroke Study Group, Cerebral sinovenous thrombosis in children. N Engl J Med 2001;345(6):417–23.

68. Heller C, Heinecke A, Junker R, et al. Cerebral venous thrombosis in children. A multifactorial origin. Circulation 2003;108:1362–7.

69. Kirton A, Shroff M, Pontigon AM, et al. Risk factors and presentations of venous infarction vs arterial presumed perinatal ischemic stroke. Arch Neurol 2010;67(7):842–8.

70. Kenet G, Lütkhoff LK, Albisetti M, et al. Impact of thrombophilia on risk of arterial ischemic stroke or cerebral sinovenous thrombosis in neonates and chil-dren: a systematic review and meta-analysis of obser-vational studies. Circulation 2010;121(16):1838–47.

71. Connor SE, Jarosz JM. Magnetic resonance imaging of cerebral venous sinus thrombosis. Clin Radiol 2002;57(6):449–61.

72. Widjaja E, Shroff M, Blaser S, et al. 2D time-of-flight MR venography in neonates: anatomy and pitfalls. AJNR Am J Neuroradiol 2006;27:1913–8.

73. Teksam M, Moharir M, Deveber G, et al. Frequency and topographic distribution of brain lesions in pediatric cerebral venous thrombosis. AJNR Am J Neuroradiol 2008;29(10):1961–5.

74. Moharir M, Shroff M, MacGregor D, et al. Clinical and radiographic features of thrombosis propaga-tion in neonatal and childhood cerebral sinovenous thrombosis. Ann Neurol 2006;60(Suppl):S141.

75. Coutinho J, de Bruijn SF, Deveber G, et al. Antico-agulation for cerebral venous sinus thrombosis. Cochrane Database Syst Rev 2011;8:CD002005.

76. Jordan LC, Rafay MF, Smith SE, et al. International Pediatric Stroke Study Group. Antithrombotic Treat-ment in Neonatal Cerebral Sinovenous Thrombosis: results of the international pediatric stroke study. J Pediatr 2010;156(5):704–10.

77. Gentilomo C, Franzoi M, Laverda AM, et al. Cerebral sinovenous thrombosis in children: throm-bophilia and clinical outcome. Thromb Res 2008; 121(4):589–91.

78. Wasay M, Dai AI, Ansari M, et al. Cerebral venous sinus thrombosis in children: a multicenter cohort from the United States. J Child Neurol 2008;23(1):26–31.

79. Berfelo FJ, Kersbergen KJ, van Ommen CH, et al. Neonatal cerebral sinovenous thrombosis from symptom to outcome. Stroke 2010;41:1382–8.

80. Kenet G, Kirkham F, Niederstadt T, et al. European Thromboses Study Group. Risk factors for recurrent venous thromboembolism in the European collaborative paediatric database on cerebral venous thrombosis: a multicentre cohort study. Lancet Neurol 2007;6:595–603.

81. Nowak-Gottl U, Junker R, Kreuz W, et al. Risk of recurrent venous thrombosis in children with combined prothrombotic risk factors. Blood 2001;97:858–62.

82. Papile LA, Burstein J, Burstein R, et al. Incidence and evolution of subependymal and intraventricular hemorrhage: a study of infants with birth weights less than 1,500 gm. J Pediatr 1978;92:529.

83. Rennie J, Hagmann CF, Robertson NJ. The baby who had an ultrasound as part of a preterm screening protocol. In: Neonatal cerebral investigation. Cambridge University Press; 2008. p. 177.

84. Larroque B, Marret S, Ancel PY, et al. White matter damage and intraventricular hemorrhage in very preterm infants: the EPIPAGE study. J Pediatr 2003;143(4):477–83.

85. Hintz SR, Kendrick DE, Wilson-Costello DE, et al. NICHD Neonatal Research Network. Early-childhood neurodevelopmental outcomes are not improving for infants born at <25 weeks' gestational age. Pediatrics 2011;127(1):62–70.

86. Kadri H, Mawla AA, Kazah J. The incidence, timing, and predisposing factors of germinal matrix and intraventricular hemorrhage (GMH/IVH) in preterm neonates. Childs Nerv Syst 2006;22(9):1086–90.

87. Del Bigio MR. Cell proliferation in human ganglionic eminence and suppression after prematurity-associated haemorrhage. Brain 2011;134:1344–61.

88. Folkerth RD. Germinal matrix haemorrhage: destroying the brain's building blocks. Brain 2011; 134:1259–63.

89. Ballabh P. Intraventricular hemorrhage in premature infants: mechanism of disease [review]. Pediatr Res 2010;67(1):1–8.

90. Ramenghi LA, Fumagalli M, Groppo M, et al. Germinal matrix haemorrhage: intraventricular haemorrhage in very-low-birth-weight infants: the independent role of inherited thrombophilia. Stroke 2011;42(7):1889–93.

91. Volpe JJ. Brain injury in the premature infant: overview of clinical aspects, neuropathology, and pathogenesis. Semin Pediatr Neurol 1998; 5(3):135–51.

92. Hagmann CF. Interobserver variability in assessment of cranial ultrasound in very preterm infants. J Neuroradiol 2011. [Epub ahead of print].

93. Maalouf EF, Duggan PJ, Counsell SJ, et al. Comparison of findings on cranial ultrasound and magnetic resonance imaging in preterm infants. Pediatrics 2001;107(4):719–27.

94. Gould DB, Phalan FC, Breedveld GJ, et al. Mutations in Col4a1 cause perinatal cerebral hemorrhage and porencephaly. Science 2005;308:1167–71.

95. Van der Knaap M, Smit LM, Barkhof F, et al. Neonatal porencephaly and adult stroke related to mutations in Collagen IV A1. Ann Neurol 2006;59:504–11.

96. De vries L, Koopman C, Groenendaal F, et al. COL4A1 Mutation in Two Preterm Siblings with antenatal onset of parenchymal hemorrhage. Ann Neurol 2009;65(1):12–8.

97. Roze E, Van Braeckel KN, Van der Veere CN, et al. Functional outcome at school age of preterm infants with periventricular hemorrhagic infarction. Pediatrics 2009;123(6):1493–500.

98. Maitre NL, Marshall DD, Price WA, et al. Neurodevelopmental outcome of infants with unilateral or bilateral periventricular hemorrhagic infarction. Pediatrics 2009;124(6):e1153–60.

99. de Vries LS, Roelants-van Rijn AM, Rademaker KJ, et al. Unilateral parenchymal haemorrhagic infarction in the preterm infant. Eur J Pediatr Neurol 2001;5:139–49.

100. Dudink J, LeQuin M, Weisglas-Kuperus N, et al. Venous subtypes of preterm periventricular haemorrhagic infarction. Arch Dis Child Fetal Neonatal Ed 2008;93(3):F201–6.

101. Lynch JK, Hirtz DG, DeVeber G, et al. Report of the National Institute of Neurological Disorders and Stroke workshop on perinatal and childhood stroke. Pediatrics 2002;109:116–23.

102. Gupta SN, Kechli AM, Kanamalla US. Intracranial hemorrhage in term newborns: management and outcomes. Pediatr Neurol 2009;40:1–12.

103. Hanigan WC, Powell FC, Miller TC, et al. Symptomatic intracranial hemorrhage in full-term infants. Childs Nerv Syst 1995;11:698–707.

104. Sachs BP, Acker D, Tuomala R, et al. The incidence of symptomatic intracranial hemorrhage in term appropriate-for-gestation-age infants. Clin Pediatr (Phila) 1987;26:355–8.

105. Armstrong-Wells J, Johnston SC, Wu YW. Prevalence and predictors of perinatal hemorrhagic stroke: results from the Kaiser Pediatric Stroke Study. Pediatrics 2009;123:823–8.

106. Brouwer AJ, Groenendaal F, Koopman C, et al. Intracranial hemorrhage in full-term newborns: a hospital-based cohort study. Neuroradiology 2010;52:567–76.

107. Hanigan WC, Powell FC, Palagallo G, et al. Lobar hemorrhages in full-term neonates. Childs Nerv Syst 1995;11:276–80.

108. Schoenberg BS, Mellinger JF, Schoenberg DG. Cerebrovascular disease in infants and children: a

study of incidence, clinical features, and survival. Neurology 1978;28:763–8.

109. Jhawar BS, Ranger A, Steven D, et al. Risk factors for intracranial hemorrhage among full-term infants: a case-control study. Neurosurgery 2003;52:581–90 [discussion: 588–90].

110. Sola MC. Evaluation and treatment of severe and prolonged thrombocytopenia in neonates. Clin Perinatol 2004;31:1–14.

111. Bergman I, Bauer RE, Barmada MA, et al. Intracerebral hemorrhage in the full-term neonatal infant. Pediatrics 1985;75:488–96.

112. Blankenberg FG, Loh NN, Bracci P, et al. Sonography, CT, and MR imaging: a prospective comparison of neonates with suspected intracranial ischemia and hemorrhage. AJNR Am J Neuroradiol 2000;21:213–8.

113. Blankenberg FG, Norbash AM, Lane B, et al. Neonatal intracranial ischemia and hemorrhage: diagnosis with US, CT, and MR imaging. Radiology 1996;199:253–9.

114. Bulas DI, Taylor GA, O'Donnell RM, et al. Intracranial abnormalities in infants treated with extracorporeal membrane oxygenation: update on sonographic and CT findings. AJNR Am J Neuroradiol 1996;17:287–94.

115. Bradley WG Jr. MR appearance of hemorrhage in the brain. Radiology 1993;189:15–26.

MR Imaging in Inflicted Brain Injury

Philippe Demaerel, MD, PhD

KEYWORDS

- MR imaging • Brain • Trauma • Nonaccidental

The estimated incidence of nonaccidental or inflicted brain injury is 0.2 in 1000 infants younger than 1 year, and is associated with a high morbidity and mortality.[1] Radiologists play an important role in the workup of suspected child abuse because the clinical presentation can be nonspecific and/or misleading. In a large series on 173 children with inflicted brain injury, 31% were initially misdiagnosed.[2] Therefore radiologists should be aware of the imaging protocol and the possible findings. Radiologists should clearly mention the possibility of nonaccidental head injury in the report whenever necessary. It cannot be sufficiently emphasized that the acute changes on imaging can be extremely subtle.

A recent systematic review investigating the features that distinguish accidental from nonaccidental injury found that apnea and retinal hemorrhages were most predictive of nonaccidental injury, followed by rib fractures.[3] Apnea leads to hypoxic-ischemic (HI) damage, and this will usually determine the outcome of the abused child.

Computed tomography (CT) is recommended as the first examination and should be performed following a cranial trauma in any child younger than 2 years.[4] Brain CT is sensitive to the detection of fresh hemorrhage and brain edema. Images at bone window setting will depict most skull fractures.

This article is limited to the role of magnetic resonance (MR) imaging in the diagnostic workup of a child with suspected inflicted brain injury.

The first issue to be addressed concerns the technique and timing of MR imaging in the workup of inflicted brain injury.

Sedation and/or general anesthesia will usually be required, and therefore the appropriate MR-compatible monitoring equipment should be available.

In addition to the standard sequences, T2-weighted, T1-weighted (fast) spin-echo, and fluid-attenuated inversion recovery (FLAIR) sequences, a T2* gradient echo sequence and a diffusion-weighted (DW) imaging sequence should always be included. Coronal and sagittal images are useful for delineating the extent of the lesions in different planes.

Three-dimensional susceptibility weighted (SW) imaging might replace T2* gradient echo sequences in the near future because of its superiority in depicting tiny hemorrhagic lesions.[5] The number and size of the hemorrhages on SW imaging appear to correlate with the neurocognitive outcome.[6] It has also been recommended to examine the cervical spine or even the whole spine, and the potential advantage of whole-body inversion recovery sequences to depict bone marrow edema is well known, although its value in inflicted brain injury remains to be proved (**Fig. 1**). In a recent article it was shown that cervical cord injury is common whereas adjacent soft-tissue injury, fractures, and dislocations are often absent.[7] The possible advantage of MR at 3 T in a child with nonaccidental intracranial injury remains to be assessed, but there seems to be a definite advantage because of the high field strength. MR venography can be used to confirm or demonstrate venous sinus thrombosis. The role of advanced MR techniques, such as MR spectroscopy, to demonstrate the presence of

The author has nothing to disclose.

Department of Radiology, University Hospital K.U.Leuven, Herestraat 49, B-3000 Leuven, Belgium

E-mail address: Philippe.Demaerel@uzleuven.be

Magn Reson Imaging Clin N Am 20 (2012) 35–44

doi:10.1016/j.mric.2011.08.007

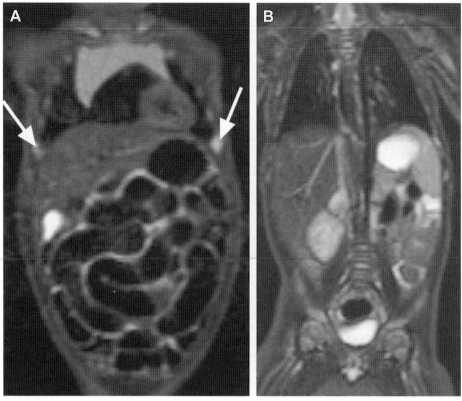

Fig. 1. (*A*) Coronal turboinversion recovery sequence of the total body shows bone marrow edema in the ribs on both sides (*arrows*). (*B*) Normal appearance of the ribs.

lactate, and diffusion tensor imaging to assess the extent of brain edema remains to be established.

It has been suggested that the ideal timing of MR imaging would be 3 or 4 days after the admission of the abused child to the emergency department.[8] A follow-up MR imaging 2 to 3 months later should be included whenever the first MR examination has demonstrated brain injury (**Fig. 2**).

Several investigators have demonstrated the contribution of MR imaging in assessing a child with suspected inflicted brain injury, and have demonstrated the superiority of MR imaging over CT in children with inflicted brain injury.[9] A recent systematic review on neuroimaging in inflicted brain injury recommends performing MR imaging in suspected head injury whenever the CT is abnormal or when there is clinical suspicion despite the normal initial CT.[10] It is well known that early signs of HI brain injury and small subdural hemorrhages can be missed on CT (**Fig. 3**). Additional information can be found on MR imaging in up to 25% of the children with abnormalities on CT.[11–13] These findings may include additional subdural hemorrhages, subarachnoid hemorrhage, axonal

shearing injury, ischemia, and contusions (**Fig. 4**). In patients with a normal CT, MR imaging was abnormal in up to 50% of cases.[10]

The authors also recommend postmortem CT and MR imaging to collect as much documentary evidence as possible for the forensic investigation. CT is more sensitive in demonstrating extracerebral hemorrhages, whereas MR imaging is superior in demonstrating parenchymal injuries (**Fig. 5**).

The second issue is the contribution of DW imaging as part of the MR imaging protocol. DW imaging is a well-established technique that adequately depicts early changes associated with restricted diffusion due to cytotoxic edema. From the literature it is clear that DW imaging plays an important role in the delineation of the extent of HI damage to the brain. In perinatal asphyxia DW imaging is the most accurate technique to demonstrate acute brain damage (**Fig. 6**). It has been suggested that an apparent diffusion coefficient value of more than 15% below the normal value ($<85 \times 10^{-5}$ mm^2/s) results in irreversible damage and a poor outcome (**Fig. 7**).[14] Whereas in adults HI lesions are usually confined to the cortex, it

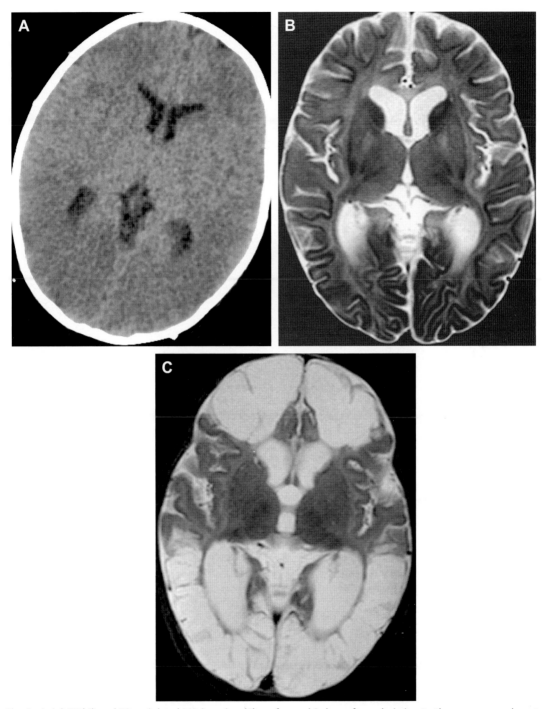

Fig. 2. Axial CT (*A*) and T2-weighted MR imaging (*B*) performed 3 days after admission to the emergency depart-ment. Follow-up MR imaging after 3 months (*C*) shows the extent of the brain damage. Brain damage is limited to the frontal and parietal watershed areas. The lesions are less clearly seen on MR image (*B*) than on CT image (*A*). The extent of the lesions is evident on the follow-up MR image (*C*).

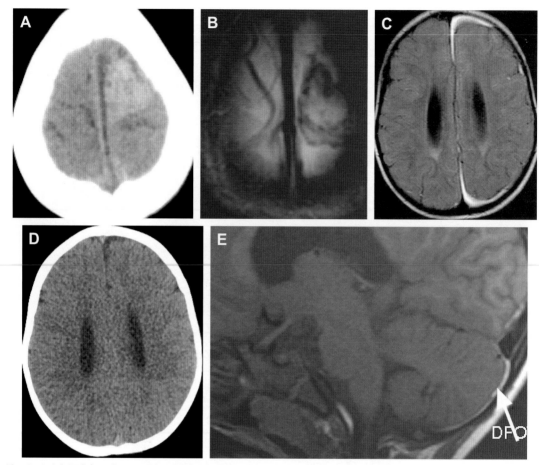

Fig. 3. Axial CT (*A*) and T2-weighted MR imaging (*B*) show a recent subdural hemorrhage on the left side close to the vertex. An additional thin subdural hemorrhage surrounding the left hemisphere is seen on FLAIR MR images (*C*) but cannot be recognized on CT (*D*). (*E*) Sagittal T1-weighted image shows another subdural hemorrhage in the posterior fossa (*arrow*).

has been demonstrated that in the term infant the parasagittal regions are involved, and in severe hypotension the putamina, thalami, hippocampi, and peri-Rolandic area are also involved (see **Fig. 6**). HI injury has also been described in the globus pallidus, another region with high metabolic demand and vascular perfusion in watershed areas. Associated damage to the pars reticularis of the substantia nigra has been observed, and has been related to anemic anoxia due to decreased hemoglobin (**Fig. 8**).[15] Pallidoreticular damage has previously been reported in carbon monoxide intoxication.[16]

The biomechanical cause of HI lesions in inflicted brain injury has not been completely elucidated. It is thought that stretching the cervical cord and lower brain stem together with squeezing the chest and strangling impairs the respiratory centers, resulting in apnea.

Several investigators have reported on DW imaging findings in inflicted brain injury. In one report on 33 children, 5 different injury patterns were found.[17] Diffuse bilateral brain swelling or brain edema limited to the watershed regions between 2 vascular territories were the most common observations (75%) (see **Fig. 7**). Venous infarction, axonal shearing injury, and focal contusion were the less common findings.

Approximately 20% of the axonal shearing injuries are only seen on DW imaging.[18]

DW imaging is extremely important because it is well known that acute HI damage can be very subtle or even undetectable on routine MR sequences (see **Fig. 2**).[19–21] In the presence of brain abnormalities on the routine MR sequences, DW imaging often demonstrates more extensive injuries.

In young children with brain injury, HI lesions occurred more frequently in nonaccidental injury

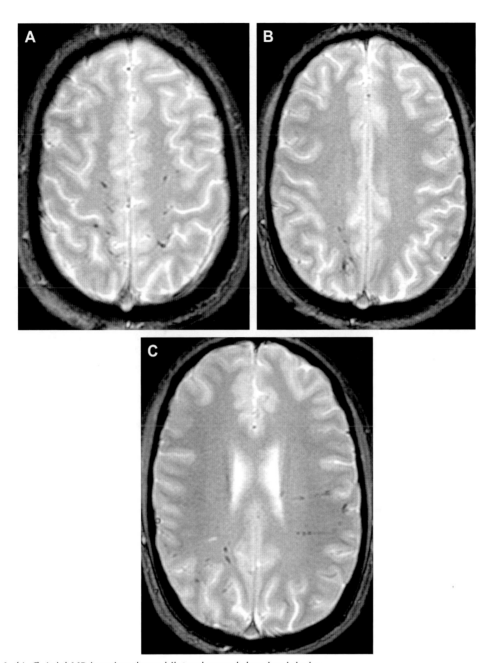

Fig. 4. (A–C) Axial MR imaging shows bilateral axonal shearing injuries.

(37%) than in accidental injury (9%).[22] It should be noted that HI injury is not limited to trauma but can also be related to anemia, drowning, hypoglycemia, and status epilepticus.

HI injury is often associated with a poor neurologic status and the need for neurosurgical intervention. The presence of HI injury and the severity of abnormalities on DW imaging correlate with a poor outcome. While HI injury usually involves both cerebral hemispheres, it has occasionally been observed to be unilateral (see Fig. 5).[23] The mechanism is not clear, but possibly shaking/strangling causes transient narrowing of the carotid artery.

It is known that subdural hematoma in an infant may appear different from subdural hematoma

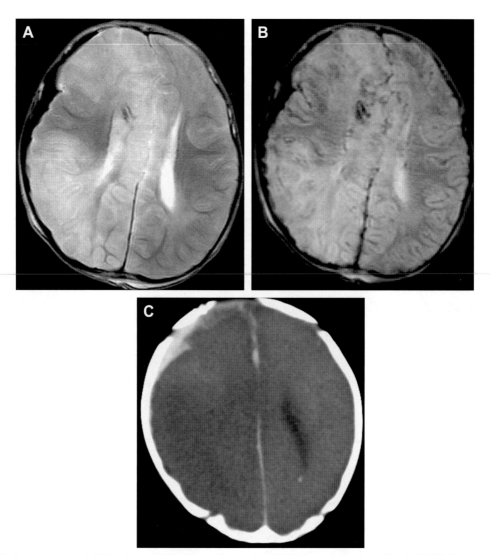

Fig. 5. Postmortem axial T2-weighted (*A*), T2* gradient echo (*B*) MR images, and axial brain CT (*C*). Parenchymal damage (both hypoxic-ischemic damage and axonal shearing injuries) is best seen on MR imaging (*A, B*) while the extra-axial hemorrhages are more clearly seen on CT (*C*). Note the unilateral distribution of the brain lesions.

later in life, and that this is influenced by the sutures, the rapidity of onset of the bleeding, and the smooth unmyelinated brain. This condition is possibly also related to the high oxygen content of the arachnoid villi, the possibility of active bleeding or rebleeding in an existing hematoma, low hematocrit, and the possible leakage of cerebrospinal fluid into the subdural hemorrhage.[24] It has been demonstrated that the forces that cause a subdural hemorrhage are greater than mere shaking, and seem to require an impact as

well.[25] While rupture of the bridging veins has been considered to be the cause of a subdural hemorrhage, new insights in the dural anatomy suggest a dural origin for the thin subdural hematoma. These bleedings within the folds of the falx might originate from endothelial damage to meningeal vessels after raised intravascular pressure.[26]

Thin subdural hematomas following parturitional trauma seem to be very common in asymptomatic newborns, particularly following instrumental delivery (**Fig. 9**).[27] This factor should be kept in

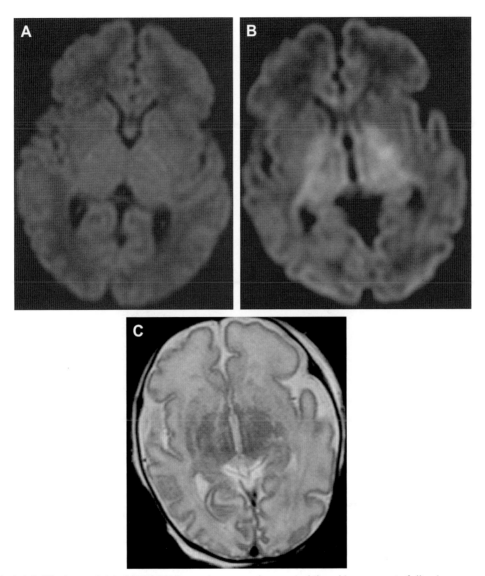

Fig. 6. Axial diffusion-weighted (DW) MR image in a normal neonate (*A*) and in a neonate following severe perinatal asphyxia (*B*). The lesions in the basal ganglia and thalami are less evident on the corresponding T2-weighted MR image (*C*).

mind when assessing brain MR imaging, and correlation with the clinical history will usually avoid further confusion.

One of the key issues in inflicted brain injury is dating the hemorrhages. Finding subdural hematomas of different age would be highly suggestive of nonaccidental injury. On CT it is accepted that a subdural hematoma is hyperdense during a period of approximately 8 days. MR imaging proved to be very accurate in dating parenchymal brain hemorrhage and therefore the expectations for dating subdural hemorrhages were very high. Unfortunately, because of the different pathophysiological environment of the subdural space, the time course of subdural hematoma is different from that of cerebral hematoma.[28] Whereas an acute parenchymal hematoma returns a low signal on T2-weighted imaging, an acute subdural hematoma returns a high signal. In the early subacute stage parenchymal hematoma remains hypointense on T2-weighted images while the subdural hematoma becomes isointense. On T1-weighted

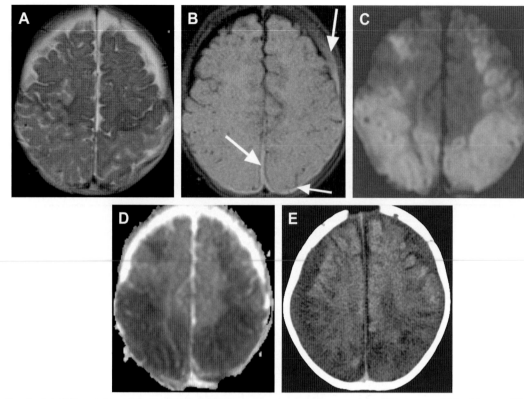

Fig. 7. Axial T2-weighted (*A*), FLAIR (*B*), DW (*C*), and corresponding apparent diffusion coefficient image (*D*) in a 5-month-old infant with hypoxic-ischemic brain injury affecting the posterior watershed areas in both parietal lobes. Follow-up CT shows the residual cortical necrosis and bilateral subdural collections (*E*). Note the presence of a (sub)dural hematoma on the left side and in the interhemispheric fissure (*B*, *arrows*).

images the early subacute subdural hematoma returns a high signal. There has been an attempt to produce a time scale, but investigators acknowledge that one should be cautious in using these data and that they cannot as such be applied in medicolegal fora.[28] There was considerable overlap between the different phases. In the acute stage, subdural hematoma appears hyperintense (supernatant) and hypointense (sediment) on T2-weighted images.

When subdural hematomas with different densities are seen on CT in different locations, it is more likely to be attributable to repeated episodes of abuse rather than to rebleeding in a preexisting hematoma.[12] The important diagnosis of repeated trauma is more difficult on MR imaging. Different signals may be observed in a reliably dated subdural bleeding, but it cannot be proved that this is rather the result of repeated trauma or spontaneous rebleeding.

MR imaging has the advantage that thin subdural or dural hemorrhages that remain undetectable on CT can be seen, and this may add useful information to the forensic investigation. It

is also likely that subdural hematomas with different intensities reflect different timing of injuries. However, it remains difficult, if not impossible, to exactly date the hematoma. Correlation with the CT and the clinical findings seems to be essential to define a time line of the nonaccidental head injury.

SUMMARY

CT is the first-line imaging procedure in a child with suspected inflicted brain injury, but MR imaging is always indicated and should preferably be carried as soon as possible, and certainly within the first 3 days. Follow-up MR imaging is recommended after 2 to 3 months.

DW imaging should always be part of the imaging protocol because of its sensitivity in detecting HI brain injury.

MR imaging is superior to CT in detecting intracranial pathology in inflicted brain injury, and this concerns brain lesions but also (sub)dural hemorrhages. Exact dating of subdural hemorrhages remains difficult even on MR imaging.

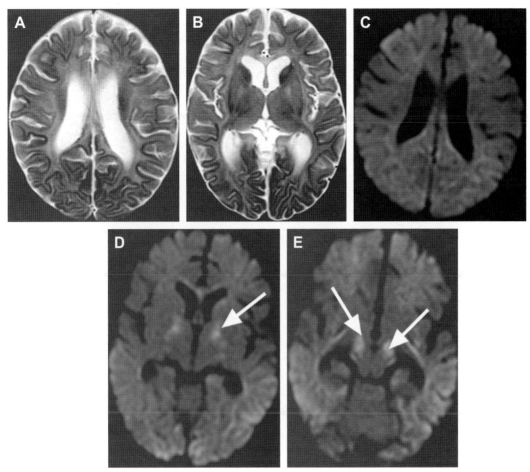

Fig. 8. Axial T2-weighted (*A, B*) and DW (*C, D*) MR images shows the predominant and bilateral involvement of the watershed areas (*C*) as well as the head of the caudate nucleus, the globus pallidus, and the substantia nigra (*D, E, arrows*). Note the poor delineation of the lesions on T2-weighted images (*A, B*).

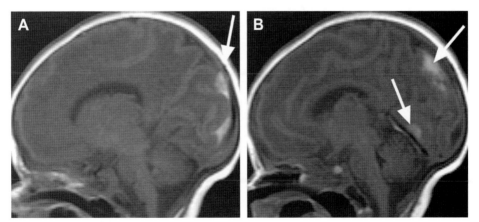

Fig. 9. Sagittal T1-weighted images (*A, B*) in a newborn after parturitional trauma shows a thin occipital and tentorial subdural hematoma (*arrows*).

REFERENCES

1. Duhaime AC, Gennarelli TA, Thibault LE, et al. The shaken baby syndrome. A clinical, pathological, and biomechanical study. J Neurosurg 1987;66:409–15.

2. Jenny C, Hymel KP, Ritzen A, et al. Analysis of missed cases of abusive head trauma. JAMA 1999;281:621–6.

3. Maguire S, Pickerd N, Farewell D, et al. Which clinical features distinguish inflicted from non-inflicted brain injury? A systematic review. Arch Dis Child 2009;94:860–7.

4. Standards for radiological investigations of suspected non-accidental injury. The Royal College of Radiologists/The Royal College of Paediatrics and Child Health 2008. Available at: http://www.rcr.ac.uk/docs/radiology/pdf/RCPCH_RCR_final.pdf. Accessed March, 2008.

5. Suskauer SJ, Huisman TA. Neuroimaging in pediatric traumatic brain injury: current and future predictors of functional outcome. Dev Disabil Res Rev 2009;15:117–23.

6. Tong KA, Ashwal S, Holshauser BA, et al. Diffuse axonal injury in children: clinical correlation with hemorrhagic lesions. Ann Neurol 2004;56:36–50.

7. Brennan LK, Rubin D, Christian CW, et al. Neck injuries in young pediatric homicide victims. J Neurosurg Pediatr 2009;3:232–9.

8. Jaspan T, Griffiths PD, McConachie NS, et al. Neuroimaging for non-accidental head injury in childhood: a proposed protocol. Clin Radiol 2003;58:44–53.

9. Foerster BR, Petrou M, Lin D, et al. Neuroimaging evaluation of non-accidental head trauma with correlation to clinical outcomes: a review of 57 cases. J Pediatr 2009;154:573–7.

10. Kemp AM, Rajaram S, Mann M, et al. What neuroimaging should be performed in children in whom inflicted brain injury is suspected? a systematic review. Clin Radiol 2009;64:473–83.

11. Ghahreman A, Bhasin V, Chaseling R, et al. Nonaccidental head injuries in children: a Sydney experience. J Neurosurg 2005;103:213–8.

12. Datta S, Stoodley N, Jayawant S, et al. Neuroradiological aspects of subdural haemorrhages. Arch Dis Child 2005;90:947–51.

13. Hoskote A, Richards P, Anslow P, et al. Subdural haematoma and non-accidental head injury in children. Childs Nerv Syst 2002;18:311–7.

14. Farina L, Bergqvist C, Zimmerman RA, et al. Acute diffusion abnormalities in the hippocampus of children with new-onset seizures: the development of mesial temporal sclerosis. Neuroradiology 2004;46:251–7.

15. Lou M, Jing CH, Selim MH, et al. Delayed substantia nigra damage and leukencephalopathy after hypoxic-ischemic injury. J Neurol Sci 2009;277:147–9.

16. Kinoshita T, Sugihara S, Matsusue E, et al. Pallidoreticular damage in acute carbon monoxide poisoning: diffusion-weighted MR imaging findings. Am J Neuroradiol 2005;26:1845–8.

17. Zimmerman RA, Bilaniuk LT, Farina L. Non-accidental brain trauma in infants: diffusion imaging, contributions to understanding the injury process. J Neuroradiol 2007;34:109–14.

18. Huisman TA, Sorensen AG, Hergan K, et al. Diffusion-weighted imaging for the evaluation of diffuse axonal injury in closed head injury. J Comput Assist Tomogr 2003;27:5–11.

19. Arbelaez A, Castillo M, Mukherji SK. Diffusion-weighted MR imaging of global cerebral anoxia. Am J Neuroradiol 1999;20:999–1007.

20. Suh DY, Davis PC, Hopkins KL, et al. Nonaccidental pediatric head injury: diffusion-weighted imaging findings. Neurosurgery 2001;49:309–20.

21. Dan B, Damry N, Fonteyne C, et al. Repeated diffusion-weighted magnetic resonance imaging in infantile non-haemorrhagic, non-accidental brain injury. Dev Med Child Neurol 2008;50:78–80.

22. Ichord RN, Naim M, Pollock AN, et al. Hypoxic-ischemic injury complicates inflicted and accidental traumatic brain injury in Young children: the role of diffusion-weighted imaging. J Neurotrauma 2007;24:106–18.

23. McKinney AM, Thompson LR, Truwit CL, et al. Unilateral hypoxic-ischemic injury in young children from abusive head trauma, lacking craniocervical vascular dissection or cord injury. Pediatr Radiol 2008;38:164–74.

24. Vinchon M, Noulé N, Jissendi Tchofo P, et al. Imaging of head injuries in infants: temporal correlates and forensic implications for the diagnosis of child abuse. J Neurosurg 2004;101:44–52.

25. Prange MT, Coats B, Duhaime AC, et al. Anthropomorphic simulations of falls, shakes, and inflicted impacts in infants. J Neurosurg 2003;99:143–50.

26. Geddes JF, Tasker RC, Hackshaw AK, et al. Dural hemorrhage in non-traumatic infant deaths: does it explain the bleeding in shaken baby syndrome? Neuropathol Appl Neurobiol 2003;29:14–22.

27. Looney CB, Smith JK, Merck LH, et al. Intracranial hemorrhage in asymptomatic neonates: prevalence on MR images and relationship to obstetric and neonatal risk factors. Radiology 2007;242:535–41.

28. Duhem R, Vinchon M, Tonnelle V, et al. Main temporal aspects of the MRI signal of subdural hematomas and practical contribution to dating head injury. Neurochirurgie 2006;52:93–104.

MR Imaging of Neonatal Spinal Dysraphia: What to Consider?

Thierry A.G.M. Huisman, MD, EQNR, FICIS[a],*,
Andrea Rossi, MD[b], Paolo Tortori-Donati, MD[b]

KEYWORDS

- Spinal dysraphism • Diastematomyelia • Neurenteric fistula
- Embryology

The development of the spinal canal and its contents is highly complex and involves multiple programmed anatomic and functional developmental and maturational processes. These processes are tightly linked to each other and interact with each other at multiple anatomic levels simultaneously.[1–3] The association of an open (non–skin covered) lumbar myelomeningocele and a Chiari II malformation is a well-known example of this multilevel interaction. In addition, malformations of the spinal canal and cord may be an isolated process involving only the neuroaxis or may be part of a complex syndrome or malformation (eg, cloacal malformation). Finally, the malformed spinal canal and cord may be secondarily injured because of prenatal, perinatal, and postnatal complications (eg, long-standing exposure of the neural tissue to the amniotic fluid, mechanical injury during delivery, or postnatal infection).

Correct and detailed knowledge about spinal malformations is essential to understand and recognize these lesions early (preferably prenatally) to counsel the parents during pregnancy, to plan possible intrauterine treatments, and to make decisions about the mode of delivery and the immediate postnatal treatment. The impact on quality of life varies significantly depending on the kind and extent of malformation. Correct classification of the identified malformation is a sine qua non. Frequently, spinal malformations are summarized as spinal dysraphism. Dysraphism is defined as an incomplete closure of a raphe or a defective fusion. Many of the malformations indeed belong to this category; however, a variety of spinal malformations may be observed that do not directly result from an incomplete closure of the neural tube during development. As two examples, early splitting of the notochord is linked to diastematomyelia (DMM), and persistence of the notochordal process may result in neurenteric fistula. Consequently, next to a detailed knowledge about the various malformations, a basic knowledge about embryology is essential.

This article discusses the imaging findings of the most frequently encountered neonatal spinal malformations and correlates these findings with the relevant embryologic processes. The presented classification is based on a correlation of clinical, neuroradiologic, and embryologic data.[1–3]

EMBRYOLOGY

The normal development of the spinal canal and its contents relies on four principal processes: (1) gastrulation with development of the notochord; (2) primary neurulation with ganglion development;

[a] Division of Pediatric Radiology, Department of Radiology and Radiological Science, Johns Hopkins Hospital, 600 North Wolfe Street, Nelson, B-173, Baltimore, MD 21287–0842, USA
[b] Department of Pediatric Neuroradiology, G. Gaslini Children's Research Hospital, Largo Gerolamo Gaslini, Genoa 1614, Italy
* Corresponding author.
E-mail address: thuisma1@jhmi.edu

Magn Reson Imaging Clin N Am 20 (2012) 45–61
doi:10.1016/j.mric.2011.08.010

(3) segmentation with appearance of the somites; and (4) secondary neurulation (caudal cell mass). These processes occur in a sequential order with partial overlap.[4–7] Based on these processes, malformations are classified as (1) disorders of primary neurulation, (2) disorders of secondary neurulation, or (3) anomalies of notochordal development.

During the first 10 to 14 days the fetus consists of two distinct cell layers: the ectoderm and endoderm (**Fig. 1**). Around the 14th day of life the process of gastrulation (Weeks 2–3) starts. Ectodermal cells glide between the endoderm and ectoderm along the primitive streak, which is localized along the craniocaudal axis of the dorsum of the embryonic disk (**Fig. 2**). During this phase the embryo transforms into a trilayered organism. Most of the cells migrate laterally between the endoderm and ectoderm to form the mesoderm. While the primitive streak is developing, it thickens at its cephalic end to form a structure called the Henson node (see **Fig. 2**). A portion of the invaginating cells remains in the midline and migrates along the craniocaudal axis of the primitive streak to form the notochordal process (see **Fig. 2**). After resorption of the floor of the notochordal process the resulting prochordal plate transforms into the definitive notochord (at 20 days) (**Fig. 3**). The definitive notochord defines the primitive axis and skeleton of the embryo and is eventually replaced by the vertebral column. It extends throughout the entire embryo and reaches as far as the level of the future midbrain, where it ends in the region of the future dorsum sella. Most importantly, the notochord induces the transformation of the overlying ectoderm into neuroectoderm with formation of the neural plate (see **Fig. 3**). The notochord secretes a protein called "sonic hedgehog," which plays a critical role in signaling the development of motoneurons. This induction of the neural plate signals the beginning of the primary neurulation (Weeks 3–4). Between Days 18 and 20 the neural plate transforms into a neural groove, which starts to close into a neural tube at Day 21 of gestation (**Fig. 4**). While the neural tube is closing, the neuroectoderm progressively detaches from the adjacent surface ectoderm and "dives" into the space between ectoderm and endoderm (**Figs. 5 and 6**). The adjacent surface ectoderm closes dorsally to the neural tube (see **Fig. 6**). At the cephalic and caudal end of the neural tube the anterior and posterior neuropore close at Day 25 of gestation. Simultaneously, cells at the border of the neuroectoderm and ectoderm detach to form the neural crests (see **Fig. 6**). The neural crests subsequently fragments and give rise to the primordial of the ganglia, which again give rise to the sensory innervations. The corresponding level of the neural tube and later spinal cord furnishes the motor innervations. A somite plate

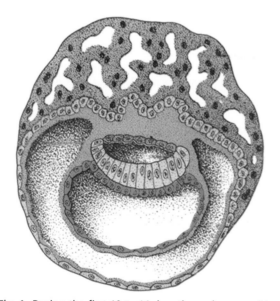
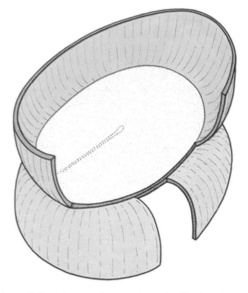

Fig. 1. During the first 10 to 14 days the embryo consists of two distinct layers: the ectoderm (*yellow*) and the endoderm (*red*). The embryonic disk is seen along the dorsum of the embryo with the developing midline primitive streak. (*From* Tuchmann-DuPlessis H, David G, Haehel P. Illustrated human embryology, embryogenesis. New York: Springer Science & Business Media (Springer-Verlag); 1982; with permission.)

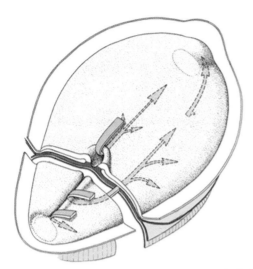

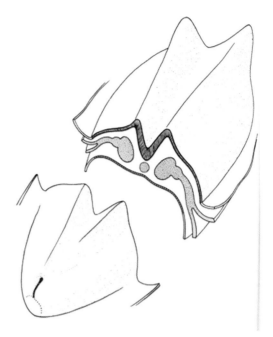

Fig. 2. During gastrulation (starting at the 14th day) the third embryonic layer, the mesoderm, forms. Around Days 15 to 16, ectodermal cells glide in the space between ectoderm and endoderm along the primitive streak. Most of the cells migrate laterally to form the mesoderm; those cells that remain in the midline migrate along the craniocaudal axis of the primitive streak to form the notochordal process. (*From* Tuchmann-DuPlessis H, David G, Haehel P. Illustrated human embryology, embryogenesis. New York: Springer Science & Business Media (Springer-Verlag); 1982; with permission.)

Fig. 4. Between Days 18 and 20 the neural plate transforms into a raised neural groove. (*From* Tuchmann-DuPlessis H, David G, Haehel P. Illustrated human embryology, embryogenesis. New York: Springer Science & Business Media (Springer-Verlag); 1982; with permission.)

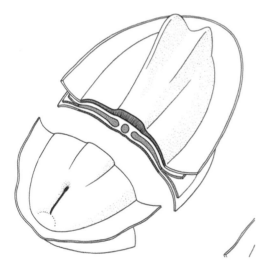

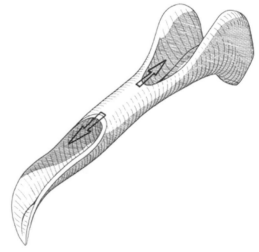

Fig. 3. During the following days the final midline notochord develops. The primary neurulation starts when the notochord induces the transformation of the overlying ectoderm into the neural plate (Day 18). (*From* Tuchmann-DuPlessis H, David G, Haehel P. Illustrated human embryology, embryogenesis. New York: Springer Science & Business Media (Springer-Verlag); 1982; with permission.)

Fig. 5. In the following days, the neural groove closes progressively while detaching from the adjacent ectoderm. In addition, the neural tube descends into the adjacent mesoderm. (*From* Tuchmann-DuPlessis H, David G, Haehel P. Illustrated human embryology, embryogenesis. New York: Springer Science & Business Media (Springer-Verlag); 1982; with permission.)

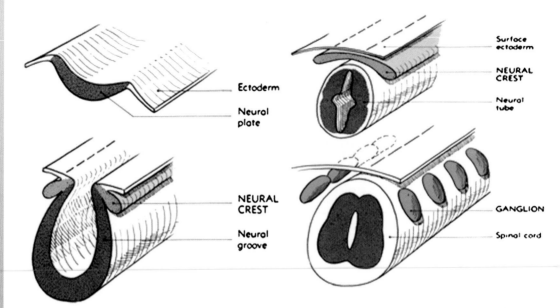

Ectoderm

Neural plate

NEURAL CREST

Neural groove

Surface ectoderm

NEURAL CREST

Neural tube

GANGLION

Spinal cord

Fig. 6. During the closure of the neural tube the overlying ectoderm closes and covers the neural tube. Simultaneously, cells at the border of the neuroectoderm and ectoderm detach and form the neural crests (*blue*). Progressive fragmentation of the neural crests gives rise to the primordial of the ganglia (*blue*). (*From* Tuchmann-DuPlessis H, David G, Haehel P. Illustrated human embryology, embryogenesis. New York: Springer Science & Business Media (Springer-Verlag); 1982; with permission.)

develops on each side of the neural tube, which also becomes segmentated (somite) (**Fig. 7**). At the end of the 5th week of gestation, 42 pairs of somites are noted (see **Fig. 7**). The somites develop a central cavity; the internal side gives rise to the sclerotome, which again migrates toward the notochord and becomes the vertebral primordial. Cells include fibroblasts, chondroblasts,

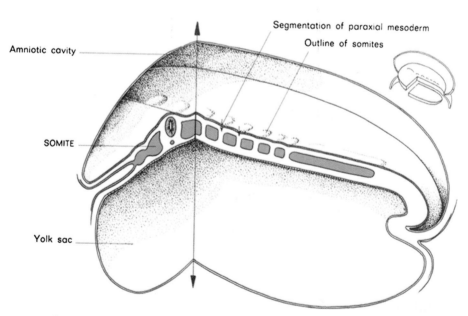

Amniotic cavity

Segmentation of paraxial mesoderm

Outline of somites

SOMITE

Yolk sac

Fig. 7. A somite plate develops on each side of the neural tube, which becomes the somites after progressive segmentation. At the end of the 5th week, 42 pairs of somites are noted. The somites further differentiate into sclerotomes, dermatomes, and myotomes. (*From* Tuchmann-DuPlessis H, David G, Haehel P. Illustrated human embryology, embryogenesis. New York: Springer Science & Business Media (Springer-Verlag); 1982; with permission.)

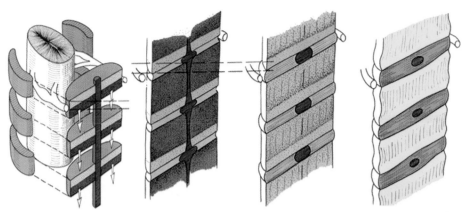

Fig. 8. The caudal half of each sclerotome joins the cephalic part of the subjacent sclerotome resulting in the intersegmental origin of the vertebral bodies. The lowest part of the cranial half of each sclerotome forms the intervertebral disk. The notochord regresses at the level of the future vertebral bodies but persists at the level of the intervertebral disks to become the nucleus pulposus. (*From* Tuchmann-DuPlessis H, David G, Haehel P. Illustrated human embryology, embryogenesis. New York: Springer Science & Business Media (Springer-Verlag); 1982; with permission.)

and osteoblasts. The part of the somite that remains in place becomes the dermomyotomes. The dermomyotomes are subsequently divided into dermatomes and myotomes. The myotomes give rise to the vertebral muscles. The caudal half of each sclerotome joins the cephalic part of the subjacent sclerotome resulting in the intersegmental origin of the vertebral bodies (**Fig. 8**). The lowest part of the cranial half of each sclerotome forms the intervertebral disk. The notochord regresses at the level of the vertebral bodies but persists at the level of the intervertebral disks and becomes the nucleus pulposus (see **Fig. 8**). The paraxial musculature

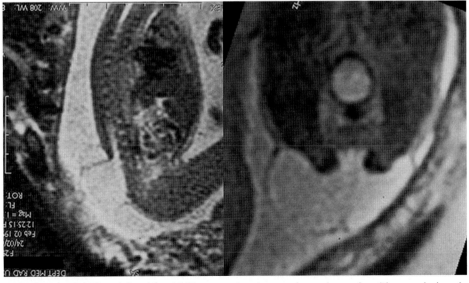

Fig. 9. Sagittal and axial T2-weighted fetal MR mages. Lumbar myelomeningocele with neural placode on top the cerebrospinal fluid filled cele. The nerve roots are seen along the ventral contour of the neural placode and appear significantly stretched on their course to the neural foramina.

derived from the somites remains segmental, allowing the musculature to bridge from one vertebral body to the next. This gives maximal flexibility and mobility of the vertebral column. The spinal nerves remain segmental and consequently leave the spinal canal between the intervertebral foramina.

Next to the primary neurulation, which is responsible for the development of the brain and upper 90% of the spinal cord, the process of secondary neurulation (Weeks 5–6) forms the lower 10% of the spinal cord and filum terminale. Secondary neurulation starts after completion of the primary neurulation and proceeds until Day 48 of gestation. Inferior to the posterior neuropore a mass of cells derived from the caudal end of the primitive streak groups together and forms the distal spinal cord by a process of canalization, retrogressive

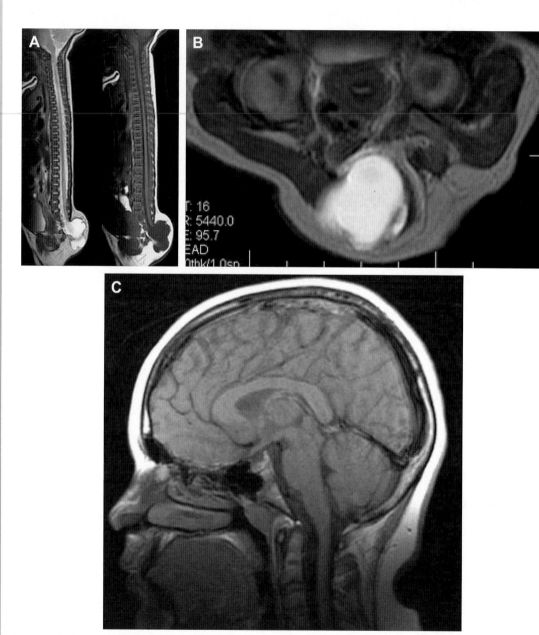

Fig. 10. Sagittal T2 and T1-weighted MR images (*A*) and axial T2-weighted MR images (*B*) of the spine in a neonate with a lipomyelomeningocele. The tethered spinal cord is protruding through a lumboscaral osseous defect into a large CSF-filled cele, which is covered by a moderate-sized subcutaneous lipoma (*A, B*). The overlying skin is closed. (*C*) No Arnold-Chiari II malformation is seen on sagittal T1-weighted MR images of the brain.

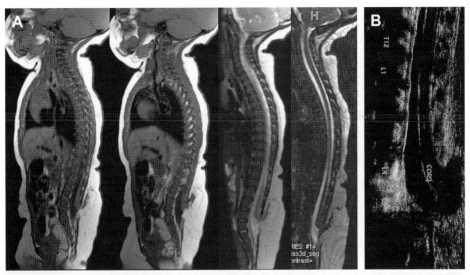

Fig. 11. Sagittal T1 and T2-weighted MR images of the spinal cord in a neonate with a lipomyelocele. (*A*) A tethered spinal cord is seen ending in a neural placode with broad attachment to a subcutaneous lipoma. No Arnold-Chiari II malformation is noted. (*B*) The matching sagittal ultrasound confirms the MR imaging findings with a tethered cord and neural placode attached to the subcutaneous lipoma.

differentiation, and finally fusion with the primary neural tube.

DISORDERS OF PRIMARY NEURULATION

From a clinical and embryologic perspective the disorders of primary neurulation can be divided into (1) open spinal dysraphia, (2) dorsal dermal sinus, and (3) closed spinal dysraphia.[1–3] In the open spinal dysraphia neural tissue is exposed to the skin with leakage of cerebrospinal fluid (CSF), whereas in the closed spinal dysraphia the malformed neural tube is covered by mesodermal (subcutaneous fat) and ectodermal (skin) elements. In these malformations no neural tissue is freely exposed and no leakage of CSF is present. In the case of a dorsal dermal sinus, a narrow canal persists between the neural tube and the overlying skin. Frequently, a small dimple is noted with intermittent leakage of drops of CSF, especially while the neonate is crying. The term "spina bifida occulta" is still en vogue but

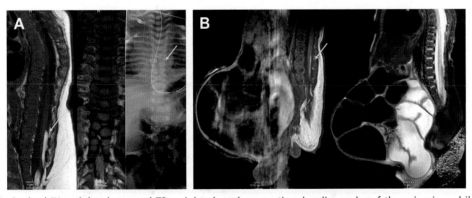

Fig. 12. Sagittal T1-weighted, coronal T2-weighted, and conventional radiography of the spine in a child with a lipomyeloceles. (*A*) T1-hyperintense intradurally extending subcutaneous lipoma (*arrow*) is noted with broad attachment to the mildly tethered spinal cord. Additional vertebral segmentation and formation anomalies (*arrow*) are noted at the thoracic level and a cardiac malformation. (*B*) Sagittal T1 and T2-weighted MR imaging of the lower abdomen reveals an anterior abdominal wall defect with bladder exstrophy (*arrow*).

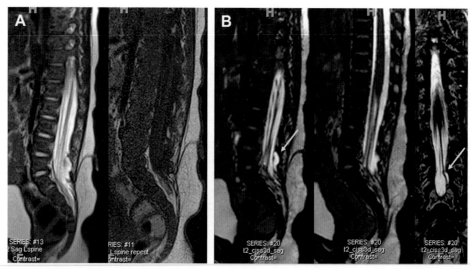

Fig. 13. Sagittal T2 and T1-weighted MR images of the lumbar spine in a neonate with a dorsal dermal sinus. (*A*) T1 and T2-hypointense sinus tract is seen coursing through the subcutaneous fat. (*B*) High-resolution, heavily T2-weighted sagittal and coronal MR image shows that the sinus tract extends intradurally and reaches the cauda equina/conus medullaris (*arrows*).

should be limited to the presence of a defective or incomplete fusion of the posterior osseous elements of the vertebral bodies. In these cases the neurulation is completed, the spinal cord is unremarkable, and the skin is covered. No associated central nervous system malformations are present. These "schisis" of the posterior vertebral arch are a frequent nonsignificant finding, predominantly involving the lumbar spine. All malformations of primary neurulation are

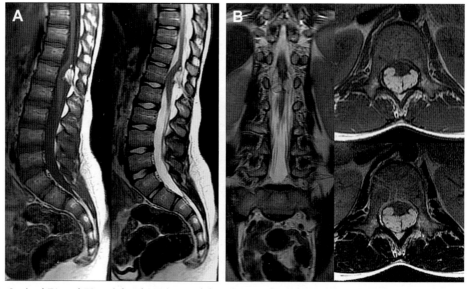

Fig. 14. Sagittal T1 and T2-weighted MR image (*A*) and coronal/axial T1-weighted MR image (*B*) of the lumbar spine in a neonate with a dorsal dermal sinus ending in an intradural lipoma. The sinus tract is seen between the spinous processes of L1 and L2, ending in a T1 and T2-hyperintense intradural lipoma, which is tightly attached to the distal lumbar spinal cord (*A*). Axial and coronal imaging shows that the spinal cord is wrapped by the lipoma (*B*).

characterized by cutaneous stigmata (birthmarks) with various degrees of skin discoloration or a hairy tuft.[8]

Open (Non–Skin Covered) Spinal Dysraphia

These malformations have the most significant impact on the quality of life for the affected child. They are classified as myelocele (MC) and myelomeningocele (MMC).[1–3] Both malformations result from a disturbance of the primary neurulation. An incomplete or segmental defective closure of the neural tube results in a neural placode that failed to detach from the adjacent surface ectoderm. Consequently, a flattened midline neural placode is either in level with the cutaneous surface (myelocele) or is pushed above or dorsal to the adjacent skin by the CSF anteriorly to the neural placode (myelomeningocele) (**Fig. 9**). Adjacent bone, muscle, and skin are also deficient in various degrees of severity. These malformations most frequently occur at the lumbar level; however, the thoracic or cervical spinal cord may also be involved. MMCs are more frequently encountered than MCs. Because the neural placode is directly exposed to the air direct surgical repair is indicated to prevent further damage or secondary inflammation of the malformed spinal cord. The neural placode itself is believed to be less functional because of multiple complex primary and secondary processes including the failure of closure itself with resulting deranged neuroarchitecture but also because of chronic injury resulting from the long-lasting exposure of the neural tissue to the amniotic fluid. In addition, all children (100%) with an open spinal dysraphia have an associated Chiari II malformation. It is believed that the chronic leakage of CSF at the level of the neural placode during the intrauterine development of the fetal brain, in particular the rhombencephalic vesicle, results in an incomplete or defective expansion of the rhombencephalic vesicle, which in turn prevents normal growth of the skull base and posterior fossa.[9] The postnatally observed anatomic features of a Chiari II malformations can at least partially be explained by a too small posterior fossa with resultant upward and downward herniation of cerebellar and brainstem structures.[9,10] In several centers around the world, based on this hypothesis open spinal dyraphias are closed as early as possible during intrauterine life with the goal to limit the severity of Chiari II malformation, in particular the degree of hydrocephalus. Identification of a MC or MMC is rather straightforward on prenatal and postnatal MR imaging (see **Fig. 9**). A midline neural placode is seen at the top of the MC or MMC either in level with the adjacent surface ectoderm or protruding above the level of the surface ectoderm. Nerve roots appear along the anterior surface of the

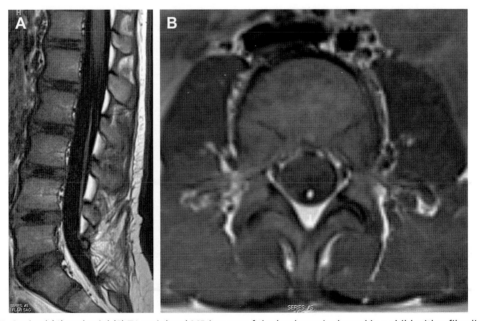

Fig. 15. Sagittal (*A*) and axial (*B*) T1-weighted MR images of the lumbar spinal canal in a child with a fibrolipoma of the filum terminale. A T1-hyperintense thickened filum terminal is seen on sagittal imaging (*A*). On axial imaging the fibrolipoma is identified as a strongly T1-hyperintense "dot" (*B*).

neural placode and depending on the degree of neural placode protrusion appear "stretched" in their course toward the neural foramina. In MMC malformations various degrees of meningeal structures are encountered herniating next to the neural placode. The spinal canal is usually widened with hypoplastic lateral and dorsal musculoskeletal derivates. Infrequently, the neural placode may protrude asymmetrically outside of the malformed spinal canal. In addition, various degrees of hydromyelia may be encountered in the intact spinal cord superior to the MC or MMC. Within the cranial vault the typical stigmata of a Chiari II malformation are encountered. All these findings should nowadays be detected by prenatal ultrasound examinations and if necessary confirmed by prenatal fetal MR imaging.[11]

Closed (Skin Covered) Spinal Dysraphism

Skin covered or closed spinal dysraphisms include lipomyeloceles (LMC) and lipomyelomeningoceles (LMMC).[1–3] These malformations have a significantly better clinical and neurologic prognosis because the neural tissue is covered and protected by skin and subcutaneous tissue. They are believed to result from a premature disjunction of the neural tube from the adjacent surface ectoderm before the neural tube is completely closed.[1–3] Consequently, mesenchymal elements of the adjacent mesoderm have access to the inner surface of the not yet completely closed neural tube. For reasons not completely understood, the interaction of mesenchymal elements with the inner lining of the neural tube induces an excess production of fat. Depending on the amount and extension of the fat, various size lipomas occur that may be located exclusively intradural or may extend into the subcutaneous region.[12–15] Because the overlying skin is closed and no CSF leakage occurs, no associated Chiari II malformation is encountered and the neural placode is less injured because of chronic exposure to the amniotic fluid during intrauterine life.

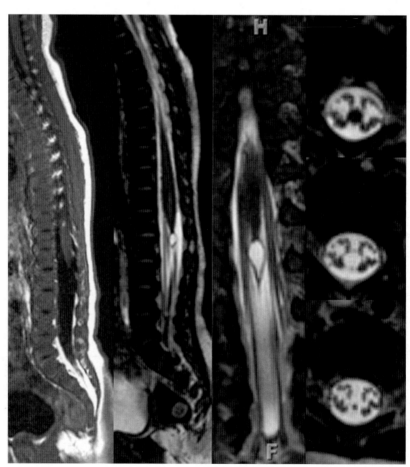

Fig. 16. Sagittal T1, thin-sliced heavily T2-weighted sagittal, coronal, and axial MR image of the lumbar spinal cord in a child with a tight filum terminal and associated CSF-filled cyst. The cyst is well demarcated, the filum mildly thickened.

Consequently, the neurologic function is preserved at a higher functional level compared with the open, non–skin covered spinal dysraphisms. Most children can walk but may suffer from bladder and bowel dysfunction.

Similar to the open spinal dysraphisms, the closed malformations are classified depending on the amount of tissue that is protruding outside of the spinal canal. If the neural tissue is seen within the level of the spinal canal the malformation is classified as LMC; if the neural tissue is pushed outside of the level of the spinal canal it is classified as LMMC (**Figs. 10** and **11**). The size of the lipoma can vary significantly and may pose a large cosmetic issue for the child, especially if the child grows older. Surgical reduction of the lipoma is frequently performed later during life.

On imaging both the LMC and LMMC are easily identified by prenatal and postnatal MR imaging examination (see **Figs. 10** and **11**). Postnatal ultrasound examination may also be a helpful bedside alternative (see **Fig 11B**). On imaging, precise

identification of the interface between the lipoma and the neural placode is essential for guiding surgical correction. The lipoma may exert massive mass effect on the neural placode, even resulting in partial rotation of the neural placode with asymmetric protrusion of meninges outside of the level of the spinal canal. In addition, the radiologist should be aware that these malformations may be associated with various other malformations (eg, cloacal malformations) (**Fig. 12**).

Dorsal Dermal Sinus

These lesions are a distinct group of malformations that seem to be an intermediate between open and closed spinal dysraphisms.[1,16–18] They consist basically of an epithelium-lined fistulous canal or tract between the skin and the adjacent spinal cord. They are believed to result from a focal or incomplete disjunction of the neuroectoderm from the surface ectoderm that is closing dorsally to the neural tube. On clinical examination, usually

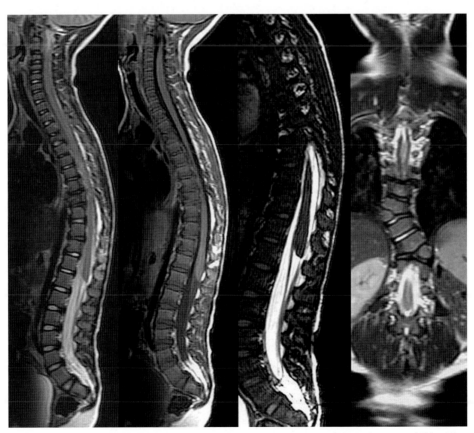

Fig. 17. Sagittal T2, T1, heavily T2, and coronal T2-weighted MR images of the spine in a child with a caudal regression syndrome. The distal sacral vertebral bodies are lacking and the distal spinal cord ends abruptly. Additional segmentation and formation anomalies are noted affecting the lower thoracic vertebral bodies.

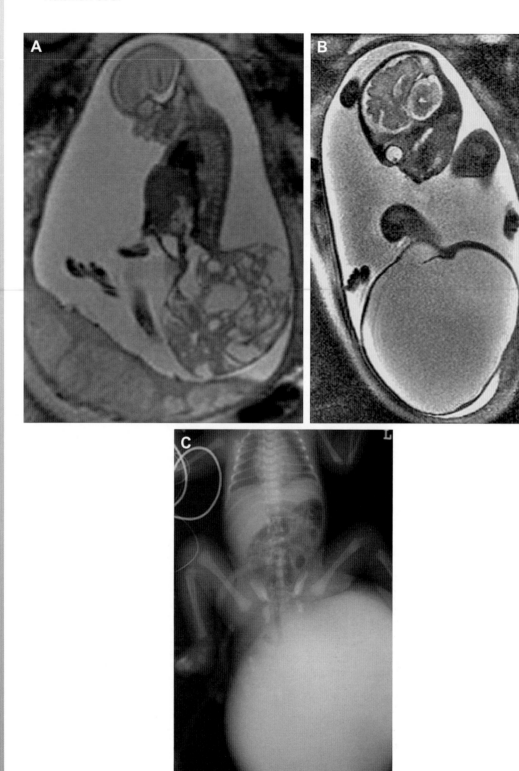

Fig. 18. Fetal MR images of two neonates with SCT. (*A*) The first neonate shows a large solid and cystic SCT, which is predominantly outside of the pelvis. (*B, C*) The second neonate shows a predominantly cystic SCT, which remained intact during cesarean delivery. The babygram (*C*) gives a good overview about the size of the SCT and the intact pelvic bones.

a midline dimple or small pin point ostium is seen from which clear CSF may intermittently leak. They represent a port of entry for infections and may result in a caudal syndrome with extensive inflammation of the radices of the cauda equine. The CSF leakage is frequently missed by parents because the neonatal diapers absorb the leaked CSF. Most dorsal dermal sinus lesions are in the lumbar region; however, thoracic and cervical cases have been described in the literature.

The fistulous tract is well seen on thin-sliced, high-resolution T1- or T2-weighted images as a T1-hypointense, T2-hypointense, or hyperintense linear streak extending from the cutaneous dimple toward the spinal cord (**Fig. 13**). The tract is usually well seen on non–fat saturated sequences because the adjacent subcutaneous fat serves gives good lesion contrast. The tract is most frequently directing upward and cranially and in up to 50% of cases ends in an intradural lipoma that is adherent to the involved segment of the spinal cord (**Fig. 14**). On very thin, heavily T2-weighted long echo imaging the fistulous tract may be directly identified between the nerve roots of the cauda equine (see **Fig. 13B**). The malformation may result in a low-lying spinal cord also known as "tethered cord." Preoperative imaging should identify the associated intradural lipoma, which has to be completely resected by the neurosurgeon to prevent recurrent spinal cord complications or recurrent cord tethering.

DISORDERS OF SECONDARY NEURULATION

Disorders of secondary neurulation affect per definition the lowest part of the spinal cord including the conus medullaris and filum terminale. Various distinct lesions may result including (1) the fibrolipoma of the filum terminale, (2) tight filum terminale syndrome, (3) caudal regression syndrome, and (4) saccrococcygeal teratoma.

Fibrolipoma of the Filum Terminale

The fibrolipoma of the filum terminale is an excess fatty infiltration of a thickened filum terminale.[1,19,20] This is a frequent normal finding on autopsy studies (4%–5%) and is only relevant if spinal cord compression or tethering occurs.

The excess fat is easily identified as a bright signal on axial or sagittal T1-weighted non–fat saturated MR imaging of the cauda equine (**Fig. 15**).

Tight Filum Terminale

This entity is characterized as a short, abnormally thick filum terminale that may result in a low-lying

(below L2), tethered conus medullaris.[1,21] It may be associated with a lipoma or infrequently with a cyst (**Fig. 16**). The thickening of the filum (>2 mm) is difficult to recognize, more importantly the tethering of the conus medullaris is seen by MR imaging.

Caudal Regression Syndrome

Caudal regression syndrome is a severe disorder with partial absence of the caudal spinal cord and matching vertebral osseous elements.[1,22–25] It involves more frequently only the secondary neurulation; however, simultaneous involvement of both the primary and secondary neurulation may occur. Caudal regression syndrome is frequently associated with various urogenital tract malformations; pulmonary hypoplasia (caused by renal insufficiency); imperforate anus; and lower limb abnormalities. In addition, caudal regression syndrome may be seen as part of the OEIS association (omphalocele, exstrophy, imperforate anus, spinal defects).

Imaging findings are characteristic with lack of the most distal segments of the spinal cord and matching musculoskeletal elements. Typically, the spinal cord abruptly terminates with a club- or wedge-shaped inferior border (**Fig. 17**). The sacrum and coccyx are typically absent. Depending on the level of affection, additional lumbar or thoracic vertebral bodies may be lacking. The malformation can be categorized into two types

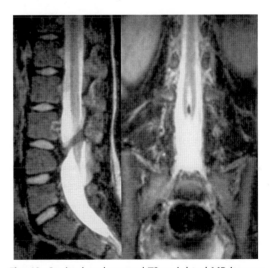

Fig. 19. Sagittal and coronal T2-weighted MR images of the lumbar spine in a child with a bony DMM. The bony spur divides the spinal canal and cord in two halves, which join inferior to the T2-hypointense bony spur. Mild hydromyelia is noted superior to the bony spur.

depending on the location and shape of the conus medullaris: either high and abrupt (type I) or low and tethered (type II). The hips are frequently dislocated and the musculature highly hypoplastic.

Sacrococcygeal Teratoma

Sacrococcygeal teratomas (SCT) are the most frequently encountered tumors in neonates.[26] They arise from the pluripotent cells of the caudal cell mass. SCT occur more often in girls than in boys (3:1 ratio). Depending on their extension SCT are classified as types I to IV. In type I the lesion is exclusively outside of the pelvis, and in type IV entirely inside of the pelvis. The large size

of the tumor may result in lethal fetal hydrops and poses a significant risk for the mother and fetus during delivery. Prenatal ultrasound and fetal MR imaging allow easy identification and characterization (cystic vs solid) of SCT (**Fig. 18**). These data guide management of pregnancy, delivery, and immediate postnatal care. Definite treatment includes complete resection of the SCT, which also requires complete resection of the coccyx to prevent recurrent tumor. Postnatal MR imaging is helpful in the preoperative diagnostic work-up to exactly delineate the extent of SCT into the pelvis and degree of displacement and infiltration of the pelvic organs. Intraspinal extension is rarely present.

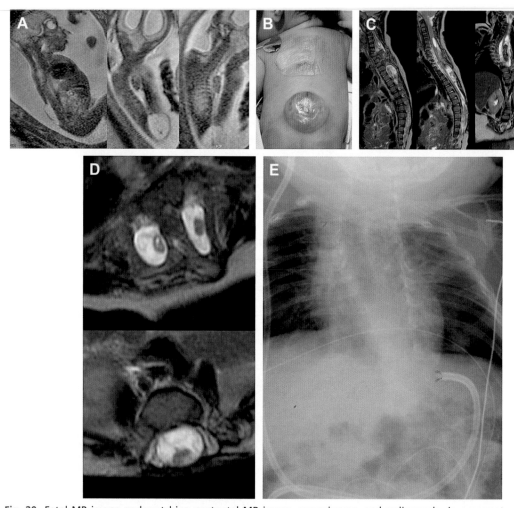

Fig. 20. Fetal MR image and matching postnatal MR image, macroimage, and radiography in a neonate with a combined thoracic DMM and lumbar MMC. (*A*) Prenatal MR image shows a large lumbar MMC and a DMM with a wide T2-hypointense bony spur dividing the spinal canal and cord in two. The spinal canal is mildly widened at the level of the DMM. (*B*) Postnatal macroimage reveal the open MMC; the DMM is covered because of a small skin laceration. Postnatal MR imaging (*C, D*) and plain radiography (*E*) confirm the prenatal imaging findings. Two hemicords are noted at the level of the DMM.

ANOMALIES OF NOTOCHORDAL DEVELOPMENT

Disorders of notochordal development are various and complex. These malformations show a partial overlap with disorders of secondary neurulation (eg, caudal regression syndrome) depending on their definition. The following malformations may be encountered: (1) split notochord syndromes also known as DMM; (2) neurenteric fistula and (3) segmental disorders of notochordal development resulting in the previously described spectrum of caudal regression syndromes; and (4) segmentation and formation anomalies of the vertebral column.

Diastematomyelia

DMM is believed to result from an abnormally widened primitive streak; the ectodermal cells that are encoded to glide between the ectoderm and endoderm consequently do not remain in the midline but form two, more laterally positioned hemi-notochord separated from each other by intervening primitive streak cells.[1,27–30] These two hemi-notochords induce the standard transformation of the overlying surface ectoderm into neuroectoderm eventually resulting into two hemicords. These hemicords may be separated from each other by either a membranous septum or a bony spur. Each final hemicord has one ventral and one dorsal nerve root and one central canal. In addition, the two hemicords may either be located within a single, shared dural sack or in two separate dural sacs. DMM is typically classified based on the encountered anatomic findings. Often associated segmentation and formation anomalies are seen affecting the vertebral bodies. DMM may involve multiple levels simultaneously but most frequently only one level is involved. Girls are more frequently affected than boys. DMM is most commonly encountered at the lumbar or thoracic level (**Fig. 19**). The overlying skin is closed but cutaneous stigmata are seen in 50% to 70% of patients; up to 90% of patients have symptoms related to cord tethering.

DMM should be diagnosed by prenatal ultrasound or fetal MR imaging (**Fig. 20**). However, short segment DMM may go undetected. Rarely, additional spinal dysraphias may be encountered, such as MMC. Postnatally, plain radiography may show a spindle-shaped, focal widening of the spinal canal on frontal projection. Bony spurs may be seen as calcified frequently "linear bars." Immediate postnatal ultrasound is a valuable and easy to perform bedside technique to study the neuroanatomy. If a surgical procedure is considered, most neurosurgeons prefer additional cross-sectional imaging including CT and

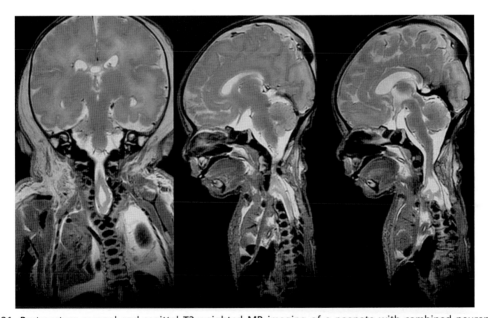

Fig. 21. Postmortem coronal and sagittal T2-weighted MR imaging of a neonate with combined neurenteric fistula and left-sided congenital diaphragmatic hernia (CDH). A T2-hyperintense band is noted extending from the anterior cervical, deformed spinal cord toward the abdominal cavity. The central canal of the spinal cord is widened, as is the spinal canal. CSF was leaking from a small pit along the anterior abdominal wall. Within the left chest cavity the dislocated spleen and bowel loops are noted, caused by the CDH.

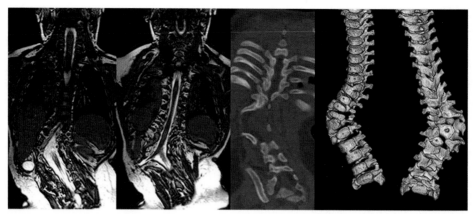

Fig. 22. Coronal heavily T2-weighted MR imaging and coronal two- and three-dimensional reconstruction of a CT examination of the spine in a child with a complex nonclassified malformation. The spinal canal appears widened at the lower thoracic level with a partial "duplication" of the distal spinal cord. The right lateral part ends in a pseudomeningocele. The CT images reveal a significant malformation of the osseous spinal canal.

MR imaging. CT is especially helpful to identify the bony spur, whereas MR imaging with thin-sliced multiplanar or three-dimensional T1- and T2-weighted sequences are most sensitive to study the exact anatomy of the spinal cord and canal. Because MMD can be multifocal, the entire spinal canal has to be studied in detail to exclude additional locations. Cord tethering is frequent; moreover, hydromyelia may coexist.[31]

Neurenteric Fistula

These malformations are extremely rare and result from a persistence of the notochordal process, which results in a direct connection between derivates of the endoderm and the neuroectoderm.[1,32,33] The spectrum of encountered findings vary widely and may include anteriorly extending neurenteric cysts and near complete sagittal extension of a fistula between the mesentery and bowel and the skin of the child's back (**Fig. 21**). These children usually suffer from severe infections because of the direct communication between contents of the spinal canal and the skin or bowel.

Segmentation and Formation Anomalies of the Spinal Column

An extensive spectrum of segmentation and formation anomalies can be encountered as (1) an incidental finding in routine chest or abdominal radiography for various reasons not related to spinal cord pathology; (2) in the diagnostic work-up of chronic back pain or progressive scoliosis; and (3) as part of various syndromes and associations (Klippel-Feil, VACTERL).[34] These hemivertebrae,

butterfly vertebrae, and block vertebrae result from a segmental derangement of the musculoskeletal somites. Identification is rather straightforward and if an orthopedic surgical intervention is considered three-dimensional CT and MR imaging should be performed to study the exact musculoskeletal anatomy and should rule out additional spinal cord anomalies. It is beyond the scope of this article to describe all possible anomalies.

SUMMARY

Many malformations present with features that seem to affect multiple developmental processes simultaneously and consequently cannot be classified in only one of the previously discussed groups of malformations (**Fig. 22**). An exact description of all findings and correlation with the embryology usually points into the direction of the predominant etiologic factor that resulted in the studied malformation. Diagnosis of spinal malformations should be done in the prenatal period (ultrasound and fetal MR imaging). Correlation of early prenatal imaging findings and postnatal studies will further increase the understanding of the intrauterine and postnatal dynamics of spinal malformations.

REFERENCES

1. Tortori-Donati P, Rossi A, Biancheri R, et al. Congenital malformations of the spine and spinal cord. In: Tortori-Donati P, editor. Pediatric neuroradiology, head, neck and spine. Berlin: Springer; 2005. p. 1552–608.
2. Tortori-Donati P, Rossi A, Cama A. Spinal dysraphism: a review of neuroradiological features with

embryological correlations and proposal for a new classification. Neuroradiology 2000;42:471–91.

3. Tortori-Donati P, Rossi A, Biancheri R, et al. Magnetic resonance imaging of spinal dysraphism. Top Magn Reson Imaging 2001;12:375–409.

4. Tuchmann-Duplessis P, David G, Heagel P. Embryogenesis. Illustrated human embryology, Vol. 1. New York: Springer; 1980. p. 19–42.

5. Tuchmann-Duplessis H, David G, Heagel P. Organogenesis. Illustrated human embryology, Vol. 2. New York: Springer; 1980. p. 2–7.

6. Nievelstein RAJ, Hartwig NG, Vermeij-Keers C, et al. Embryonic development of the mammalian caudal neural tube. Teratology 1993;48:21–31.

7. Catala M. Genetic control of caudal development. Clin Genet 2002;61:89–96.

8. Drolet B. Birthmarks to worry about. Cutaneous markers of dysraphism. Dermatol Clin 1998;16: 447–53.

9. McLone DG, Knepper PA. The cause of Chiari II malformation: a unified theory. Pediatr Neurosci 1989; 15:1–12.

10. Naidich TP, McLone DG, Fulling F. The Chiari II malformation. Part IV. The hindbrain deformity. Neuroradiology 1983;25:179–97.

11. Huisman TA. Fetal magnetic resonance imaging. Semin Roentgenol 2008;43:314–36.

12. Naidich TP, McLone DG, Mutleur S. A new understanding of dorsal dysraphism with lipoma (lipomyeloschisis): radiological evaluation and surgical correction. AJNR Am J Neuroradiol 1983;4:103–16.

13. Pierre-Kahn A, Zerah M, Renier D, et al. Congenital lumbosacral lipomas. Childs Nerv Syst 1997;13: 298–334.

14. Knittle JL, Timmers K, Ginsberg-Fellner F, et al. The growth of adipose tissue in children and adolescents. Cross-sectional and longitudinal studies of adipose cell number and size. J Clin Invest 1979; 63:239–46.

15. Catala M. Embryogenesis. Why do we need a new explanation for the emergence of spina bifida with lipoma? Childs Nerv Syst 1997;13:336–40.

16. Scotti G, Harwood-Nash DC. Congenital thoracic dermal sinus: diagnosis by computer assisted metrizamide myelography. J Comput Assist Tomogr 1980;4:675–7.

17. Barkovich AJ, Edwards MS, Cogen PH. MR evaluation of spinal dermal sinus tracts in children. AJNR Am J Neuroradiol 1991;12:123–9.

18. Weprin BE, Oakes WJ. Coccygeal pits. Pediatrics 2000;105:E69.

19. Brown E, Matthes JC, Bazan C, et al. Prevalence of incidental intraspinal lipoma of the lumbosacral spine as determined by MRI. Spine 1994;19:833–6.

20. Uchino A, Mori T, Ohno M. Thickened fatty filum terminale: MR imaging. Neuroradiology 1991;33: 331–3.

21. Yundt KD, Park TS, Kaufman BA. Normal diameter of filum terminale in children: in vivo measurement. Pediatr Neurosurg 1997;27:257–9.

22. Duhamel B. From the mermaid to anal imperforation: the syndrome of caudal regression. Arch Dis Child 1961;36:152–5.

23. Currarino G, Coln D, Votteler T. Triad of anorectal, sacral, and presacral anomalies. AJR Am J Roentgenol 1981;137:395–8.

24. Nievelstein RA, Valk J, Smit LM, et al. MR of the caudal regression syndrome: embryologic implications. AJNR Am J Neuroradiol 1994;15:1021–9.

25. Barkovich AJ, Raghavan N, Chuang SH. MR of lumbosacral agenesis. AJNR Am J Neuroradiol 1989;10:1223–31.

26. Tortori-Donati P, Rossi A, Biancheri R, et al. Tumors of the spine and spinal cord. In: Tortori-Donati P, editor. Pediatric neuroradiology, head, neck and spine. Berlin: Springer; 2005. p. 1637–8.

27. Pang D, Dias MS, Ahab-Barmada M. Split cord malformation. Part I. A unified theory of embryogenesis for double spinal cord malformations. Neurosurgery 1992;31:451–80.

28. Breningstall GN, Marker SM, Tubman DE. Hydrosyringomyelia and diastematomyelia detected by MRI in myelomeningocele. Pediatr Neurol 1992;8: 267–71.

29. Pang D. Split cord malformation. Part II. Clinical syndrome. Neurosurgery 1992;31:481–500.

30. Naidich TP, Harwood-Nash DC. Diastematomyelia. Part I. Hemicords and meningeal sheaths. Single and double arachnoid and dural tubes. AJNR Am J Neuroradiol 1983;4:633–6.

31. Schlesinger AE, Naidich TP, Quencer RM. Concurrent hydromyelia and diastematomyelia. AJNR Am J Neuroradiol 1986;7:473–7.

32. Rufener SL, Ibrahim M, Raybaud CA, et al. Congenital spine and spinal cord malformations: pictorial review. AJR Am J Roentgenol 2010;194:S26–37.

33. Menezes AH, Traynelis VC. Spinal neurenteric cysts in the magnetic resonance imaging era. Neurosurgery 2006;58:97–105.

34. Wax JR, Watson WJ, Miller RC, et al. Prenatal diagnosis of hemivertebrae: associations and outcomes. J Ultrasound Med 2008;27:1023–7.

MR Imaging of the Newborn: A Technical Perspective

Claudia M. Hillenbrand, PhD[a], Arne Reykowski, PhD[b],*

KEYWORDS

- Neonate • Magnetic resonance imaging • MR safety
- MR-compatible Incubator • NICU MR imaging
- Newborn RF coil

The demand for magnetic resonance (MR) imaging of severely compromised term and preterm infants in neonatal intensive care units (NICUs) is increasing worldwide because MR imaging, with its excellent image quality, has unequaled diagnostic and prognostic value.[1–5] MR imaging is indicated for neonates with brain injuries and neurologic disorders. In these cases, MR imaging detects more abnormalities, and shows their position and extent more precisely, than cranial ultrasound, the safe first-line imaging modality readily available in neonatal nurseries.[6–9] A recent retrospective study on 129 neonatal MR imaging examinations found that the initial ultrasound diagnosis was changed or further specified in more than 57% of patients, and MR-based changes in clinical management were initiated in 58% of patients.[4] Recent advances in MR imaging techniques add to the demand for MR imaging, because it concurrently provides quantitative structural, functional (ie, perfusion and diffusion), and vascular information. MR imaging is still a relatively new technique for imaging the newborn, and very preterm infant in particular, and an active area of research and development. Because scan duration and safety of the often critically ill infants is essential, special emphasis is placed on the development of a safe and quick imaging workflow. Therefore, improvements in equipment (ie, MR-compatible patient monitoring units, incubators, transport systems, dedicated pediatric radio frequency (RF) antennas, and so forth) and MR sequences (ie, parallel imaging and motion-correction methods) are of interest and are often worked on in tandem.

This article reviews the particular needs, equipment, and techniques for MR imaging of the newborn infant and seeks to give an outlook on future technology-driven developments in this area of research.

PRACTICAL ISSUES
Risks Associated with Neonatal MR Imaging

Most neonate MR imaging examinations are clinically indicated by injuries and malformations of the brain and spine, such as hypoxic ischemic brain injuries, seizures, trauma, inflicted head injuries, spinal dysraphia, or metabolic diseases, followed by congenital cardiac defects, cardiovascular malformations, and by musculoskeletal indications. All these applications deal with relatively unstable infants, and special management is needed to perform the scan without harming the infant. Potential hazards are acoustic noise, adverse thermal conditions, hemodynamic or ventilation instability, and general risks related to transport and handling.[4] Therefore, close and reliable monitoring of vital functions, support for respiratory and cardiovascular functions, as well as fluid electrolyte and thermoregulatory homeostasis throughout the examination, are warranted.[10] Additional risk factors are sedation or general anesthesia, which can lead to acute and long-term complications.[11] Because the MR examination by itself bears a risk to the ill and unstable

[a] Division of Translational Imaging Research, Department of Radiological Sciences, St Jude Children's Research Hospital, 262 Danny Thomas Place, Memphis, TN 38105, USA
[b] Research and Predevelopment, Invivo Corporation, Gainesville, FL 32608, USA
* Corresponding author.
E-mail address: arne.reykowski@philips.com

Magn Reson Imaging Clin N Am 20 (2012) 63–79
doi:10.1016/j.mric.2011.10.002

infant, comprehensive practice parameters and recommendations have been published for preterm and full-term neonates that specifically address the necessity and timing of the MR examination as a function of the clinical condition of the infant.[1,2,6]

MR Safety and Screening

When MR imaging is clinically indicated, the critically ill preterm or term infant usually has to be transported to the MR suite of the radiology department, which in many institutions is far from the NICU. The logistics of transport and imaging are complex and need to be carefully planned.[12] Neonatology staff (ie, NICU nurses and neonatologists experienced in neonatal resuscitation), a respiratory therapist for infants on ventilator support, and radiology staff (ie, MR technologist, MR nurse, and radiologist) need to communicate and cooperate at all times to ensure a safe preparation, transport, and examination.[1] It is important for all involved personnel to be trained in and follow MR safety guidelines, because the strong static magnetic fields and the alternating RF fields constitute MR imaging–specific risks that mandate precautions. The risk associated with the static magnetic field is not limited to the patient and extends to any person (eg, health care professional or accompanying family member) who enters the magnet room. The American College of Radiology (ACR) has published extensive guidelines on MR safety.[13] The safety recommendations by Stokowski and colleagues[14] and Benavente-Fernandez and colleagues[15] highlight issues that are particularly important and relevant to newborn infants.

It is of utmost importance to ensure that no ferrous objects are brought accidentally into the magnet room, where they could become projectiles because of the strong forces of the magnetic field. However, nonmagnetic metals can also be subject to undesired Lenz forces and torque effects, either caused by fast switching gradients or as a result of being moved inside the static magnetic field.[13] Furthermore, the combination of strong magnetic fields and high level of RF power may cause electronic equipment to fail. For these reasons, everybody needs to be screened for metal on or inside the body, including implants and pacemakers, before entering the MR scan room.[13] Common practice requires that screening forms be completed for each individual as part of the screening process.[16] An increasing number of MR imaging sites follow ACR recommendations on the use of ferromagnetic screening devices as an additional safety layer. These devices may be of particular advantage in a setting such as newborn imaging, wherein a large number of

individuals and additional equipment has to enter the magnet room.

Equipment used in the scan room should be labeled according to the scheme proposed by the US Food and Drug Administration (FDA)[13,17,18]:

MR safe: A square green "MR safe" label indicates that the item is safe to use in the MR environment and poses no known hazard; such items are nonmetallic, nonmagnetic, and nonconducting, such as plastics or wood.

MR conditional: A triangular yellow "MR conditional" label represents items that have been tested and shown to pose no known hazards in a specified MR environment (eg, maximum static magnetic field, gradients, specific absorption ratio [SAR]) in specified conditions of use (eg, certain routing of cables and leads for equipment).

MR unsafe: MR-unsafe items are labeled with a red circle with diagonal red bar, and represent items that are known to pose a clear and direct threat to persons and equipment in the scanner room (ie, ferromagnetic objects) and therefore must not be brought in.

Well-designed magnet rooms have wave guides (wall openings) between the scan room and the operator room, where fiber optic leads, plastic tubes, and other nonconducting leads or hoses can be fed through. The local MR imaging service may help identify wave guides between the technical room and the scan room. These openings enable the use of non–MR-safe monitoring equipment by placing it outside the magnet room and using fiber optics to connect to the patient. No electrically conductive leads should run through these wave guides, because they act as antennas, compromise the RF shielding of the magnet room, and lead to MR image artifacts.

RF Exposure

During a scan, the patient, as well as all the equipment, inside the MR imaging magnet bore are exposed to high-frequency RF fields. Therefore, all cables and electrically conductive materials can potentially act as antennas and attract RF currents. This can lead to tissue heating due to local hot spots in the RF transmit field in the proximity of the equipment and also to elevated surface temperatures of these items. All items inside the MR imaging bore, as well as in the vicinity, have to be specifically designed and tested for safe use inside the RF transmit field of the scanner.

As additional precautions, cables should always be placed away from the patient and run in straight lines and along the shortest route outside of the bore without forming loops. All manufacturer warnings and recommendations should be followed. Any equipment or conductive material that is not needed or not used during the scan should be removed before the examination. All devices used have to be plugged in properly to ensure safe performance. Equipment should not be used if a visual inspection reveals loss of integrity in electrical or thermal insulation.

The RF power applied to the patient is measured as SAR in Watts per kilogram (W/kg). Limits of SAR depend on many factors such as patient age, patient weight, location of patient inside the RF field, and local regulatory legislation.[19,20] In the United States, the maximum allowable SAR is 3 W/kg (averaged over 10 minutes) for head imaging and 4 W/kg (averaged over 15 minutes) for whole-body imaging.[21] To ensure that SAR limits are not exceeded, the MR imaging machine uses a so-called SAR monitor, which correlates information about MR imaging coils, patient weight, and patient position with real-time measured data relating to RF field and RF power. Because MR imaging scanners are primarily built for adult-size patients, pediatric imaging with its much smaller and lighter patients constitutes a challenge for the underlying SAR model. The user has to ensure that correct patient SAR parameters are entered into the system. It is also advisable to consult the operator's manual before using coils such as adult head coils, which have not been specifically designed for use with neonates. In some instances, scanners use the information regarding the type of local coil to estimate patient position. It is therefore always advisable to keep MR imaging coils in their intended location on the patient table.

Patient Preparation, Transportation, and Monitoring

As mentioned earlier, the logistics of transporting newborn infants from the NICU to the MR suite and the MR imaging examination are complex and need to be planned carefully. The workflow varies depending on the severity of the illness, the need for sedation, and the availability of an MR-conditional incubator. Detailed guidelines on how to prepare the unsedated critically and noncritically ill infant in the NICU for transport and MR imaging, as well as a list of equipment needed (also see **Table 1**), are given by Mathur and colleagues.[1] For an alternative description of these aspects, including sedation, the reader is referred to van Wezel-Meijler and colleagues,[2] Pennock,[16] and Maalouf and colleagues.[22]

Preparing neonates for MR imaging, whether sedated or unsedated, includes reconnecting the infant to an array of MR-safe or MR-conditional monitoring sensors such as electrocardiogram (ECG), SpO2, noninvasive blood pressure (NIBP), temperature, and respiratory sensors.[23] In addition, an MR-compatible ventilator as well as infusion pumps may be used. The patient needs to be protected from noise and must be kept warm during transport and scanning by using sheets, blankets, and maybe also a Porta-Warm infant mattress. Furthermore, patient stabilization devices are needed to reduce motion during the scan. For this purpose, vacuum cushions, foam pads, and straps may have to be applied.[1,16] Even without sedation, the preparation time for neonates is 30 to 60 minutes.

The main steps and equipment used for transportation of neonates to the MR room are as follows.

Ventilation
A ventilated infant should be transferred to an MR-compatible ventilator with MR-conditional gas cylinders before leaving the NICU. MR-compatible ventilators are available from several manufacturers (see **Table 1**). Alternatively, standard neonatal ventilators can be used. However, they need to be placed outside the magnet room with the extended hoses fed through the wave guide on the filter plate in the MR room.[2]

Intravenous solutions and pumps
The number of intravenous (IV) solutions that need to be administered during MR imaging should be minimized to the absolutely necessary before transport, and IV pumps should be exchanged with MR-compatible pumps, which are available from several manufacturers (see **Table 1**). As with non–MR-safe ventilators, non–MR-safe IV pumps can still be used, but the IV lines need to be extended and fed through the wave guide into the control area outside the scanner room where the IV pumps have to be placed.

Oxygen and heart rate
An MR-compatible pulse oximeter (see **Table 1**), with the probe preferably taped to a foot, should be used to monitor the infant's oxygen saturation level. Pulse oximeters scan the pulsatile arterial blood during each cardiac cycle to calculate the oxygen saturation, thereby also delivering data about the pulse rate and cardiac output. Hence, pulse oximeters are not only useful to detect hypoxemia and hypoxia but also to measure the real-time heart rate to detect bradycardia and apnea,[23,24] which may occur particularly in

Table 1
MR-compatible equipment needed for newborn MR imaging

Equipment	Manufacturer	Location
MR-compatible ventilator (with CPAP mode)	Airon	Melbourne, FL
	Allied	St Louis, MO
	Bio-Med Devices	Guilford, CT
	Draeger Medical	Telford, PA
	Smiths Medical	Dublin, OH
	SREE Medical Systems/Advanced Imaging Research	Cleveland, OH
	VersMed/GE	Piscataway, NJ
MR-compatible infusion pumps (intravenous pumps)	IRadimed	Winter Park, FL
	Mammendorfer Institut für Physik und Medizin	Mammendorf, Germany
	MEDRAD	Warrendale, PA
MR-compatible pulse oximeter with an infant SpO$_2$ sensor	Invivo	Orlando, FL
	Memmendorfer Institut für Physik und Medizin	Mammendorf, Germany
	MEDRAD	Warrendale, PA
	Nellcor/Covidien	Boulder, CO
	Nonin	Plymouth, MN
MR-compatible ECG leads	Conmed	Utica, NY
	Invivo	Orlando, FL
	Medicotest/Ambu	Glen Burnie, MD
Head-stabilizing equipment	CFI Medical Solutions	Flint, MI
	Par Scientific	Houston, TX
Ear protection (ear muffs)	3M	St Paul, MN
	Natus	San Carlos, CA
Portable infant warmer	3M	St Paul, MN
	Cardinal Health	Dublin, OH
	Embrace	San Francisco CA
Temperature monitoring	LumaSense Technologies	Santa Clara, CA
Neonatal RF coil	Invivo	Orlando, FL
	Lammers Medical Technology	Lübeck, Germany
	Philips	Best, Netherlands
	SREE Medical Systems/Advanced Imaging Research	Cleveland, OH
MR-conditional incubator	Koala System AB	Waxholm, Sweden
	Lammers Medical Technology	Lübeck, Germany
	SREE Medical System/Advanced Imaging Research	Cleveland, OH

Disclaimer: List represents all equipment/manufacturers known to the authors and may not be complete.
Abbreviations: CPAP, continuous positive airway pressure; ECG, electrocardiogram.

preterm infants.[1] Furthermore, MR-compatible ECG leads (see **Table 1**) may be attached to the infant's chest before leaving the NICU, to monitor the heart rate more accurately during the MR examination. Monitoring the heart rate during MR imaging is important, because changes to the heart rate have been observed in newborns and linked to the MR examination.[25,26]

Ear protection

When imaging neonates, noise reduction is essential to protect their sensitive ears from the excessive noise emanating from the MR imaging scanner. Therefore, earplugs and neonatal ear muffs (see **Table 1**) are fitted before the transport. In addition, lightweight headphones may be placed over the muffs in the MR room to further reduce noise.[2]

Temperature

It is important to monitor and maintain the body temperature of the infant during transport and MR imaging. Infant blankets used for a firm swaddle and/or a portable infant warmer together with a warming pad should be used to ensure that the infant stays warm. An MR-compatible fluoro-optic temperature probe (see **Table 1**) should be taped in the NICU to the infant's abdomen for constant monitoring of body temperature.[1,2]

Resuscitation equipment

MR-compatible resuscitation equipment should be available during transport and MR examination, including an MR-compatible laryngoscope and endotracheal tubes in various sizes suitable for newborns and a self-inflating AMBU bag. During the MR imaging examination, the resuscitation cart should be kept outside. There should also be a positive-pressure oxygen delivery system and wall suction available outside in close proximity to the MR suite.[1,2] In an emergency, any resuscitation attempt should be made outside the MR room, because the risk of an accident due to MR unsafe equipment rushed into the room during resuscitation is high.[27]

Incubator

A relatively safe transport of the infant to the MR suite and MR examination is assisted by the use of an MR-compatible incubator with integrated MR-compatible monitoring equipment and neonatal MR coils. In the NICU, the infant is placed into the incubator; earmuffs are attached; intravenous infusions, ventilators, and all necessary MR-compatible monitors are connected; and the RF coils (eg, head or body array) are attached before the infant is transferred to the MR room and scanned within the incubator. Besides offering a safe humidity-controlled and temperature-controlled environment to the infant at all times, the MR-compatible incubator optimizes the workflow because there is no additional transfer of the infant necessary when entering and leaving the MR room.

A commercially available solution, the FDA-approved LMT nomag IC 1.5/3.0 MR-conditional incubator (Lammers Medical Technology, Lübeck, Germany) with integrated MR head coil and optional body array, MR-compatible ventilation, and integrated monitoring has been installed in more than 50 centers worldwide.[28] One of the first incubators of this type was installed at the Children's Hospital in Los Angeles (**Fig. 1**)[29,30] and has been used since for ground-breaking work in structural and functional MR imaging, diffusion, and spectroscopy there[9] and in other institutions.[4,31]

Custom solutions include the incubator[32] used by the University of California San Francisco to perform pioneering work in neonatal MR imaging and spectroscopy (**Fig. 2**).[33] This incubator was built around a GE Signa patient table and docked directly to the magnet, thereby eliminating the need for lifting the incubator with the infant inside onto the patient table, in contrast with the LMT incubator, which fits all vendor platforms (eg, GE, Philips, Siemens) but requires lifting. Also, the incubator volume is approximately 3 to 4 times that of the LMT, offering more space for the infant. Other features include a closed-circuit infrared TV camera to monitor the baby, even in total darkness; double walls for added insulation and noise reduction; a massive battery bank that warrants full operation for several hours independent of wall power; thermal management hardware (controller, fan, heating elements, and so forth) that is separated from the incubator and stays outside the magnet; a filling factor optimized birdcage head coil that easily slides out of the way without moving the baby; an alternative mechanism to slide the baby into the incubator without moving the coil; and a preparation area with work lights to prepare the infant for the transport and scan.

If an MR-compatible incubator is not available, a standard transport incubator can be used. However, because the transport incubator is usually MR unsafe, the infant needs to be taken out of the incubator outside the scanner room. It is important that all equipment that is not MR safe is clearly labeled and all involved staff members are instructed to leave MR-unsafe equipment outside the magnet room.

Sedation

Sedation is usually unnecessary for newborn infants undergoing MR imaging, because most infants sleep through the examination after being properly fed, swaddled, and prepared for the scan.[1,2,34] In the few neonates who require sedation to prevent motion artifacts, orally administered chloral hydrate is frequently used.[2,16,29,35–39] An initial dose of 50 mg/kg for infants younger than 3 months is common, but dose levels vary from 25 to 55 mg/kg among institutions.[2,16,29,35–39] Institutional guidelines are usually in place for the selection and administration of effective and safe sedation during radiological procedures.[40,41]

Immediate risks introduced by chloral hydrate sedation, such as postsedation apnea, bradycardia, and oxygen desaturation, are associated with disease and indirectly associated with age, and hence are higher in very young and critically ill neonates.[38] Recent concerns have been raised about potential long-term effects such as neurodegeneration, with possible cognitive and behavioral problems.[11,42] These concerns are based on observations of neurotoxicity of anesthetic agents that show subtle, but prolonged, behavioral

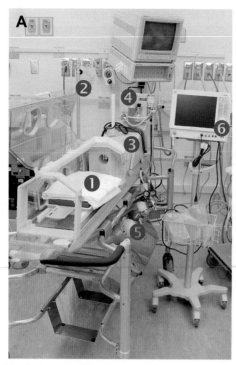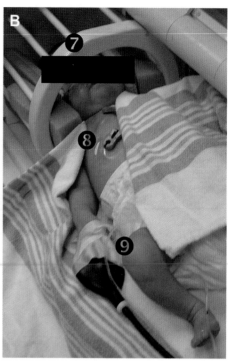

Fig. 1. The MR-compatible incubator (Lammers Medical Technology, Lübeck, Germany) used for MR imaging studies in preterm and term neonates at Children's Hospital of Los Angeles. (*A*) Overview of the incubator and necessary equipment: (**1**) infant station, (**2**) pole for IV pumps and fluids, (**3**) unit for control and regulation of temperature and humidity inside the incubator, (**4**) MR-compatible ventilator, (**5**) nonmagnetic O_2 and air supply, (**6**) MR-compatible transport monitor. (*B*) Infant placed inside the incubator in the neonate head coil (SREE Medical Systems, Cleveland, OH) (**7**) with attached ECG leads (**8**), and a deflated stimulation rubber bulb (**9**) in the unfolded palm of the right hand. Rubber bulbs in both hands are used in functional MR imaging experiments for passive stimulation (eg, inflating and deflating the bulb opens and closes the fist).[30] (*Courtesy of* Dr S. Blüml, Children's Hospital of Los Angeles.)

changes in rodent models.[42] However, the current evidence is insufficient to recommend substantial changes in clinical practice. Nevertheless, avoiding unnecessary sedation in these patients is recommended. Some institutions have therefore developed procedures and guidelines for MR imaging in neonates without giving sedation, and have been successful in consistently performing safe and high-quality MR examinations by following these procedures.[1,2,43]

RF COILS FOR NEONATAL MR IMAGING
Maximizing Signal-to-Noise Ratio

Anatomic structures are significantly smaller in infants than in adult patients. For instance, the size of the brain of an average-weight term newborn is approximately 25% that of an average adult[44,45]; higher-resolution scans are therefore needed to depict anatomic features in detail. A high signal-to-noise ratio (SNR) is a prerequisite for the increased resolution needed for MR

imaging of newborns. SNR is directly proportional to the voxel size: reducing the voxel in all 3 dimensions by 20% decreases the voxel volume and hence the SNR by approximately 50%.[46,47] Doubling the resolution in all 3 spatial dimensions results in an eightfold reduction in the voxel volume and SNR.

A potential source for additional SNR is the RF receive coil used for imaging. In many sites, adult head or extremity coils are used for scanning infants because of the lack of dedicated neonatal head or body coils.[1,2,48] Often, the size of these adult patient coils is significantly larger than that required for infants, which leads to a suboptimal filling factor.[49] The filling factor is a figure of merit for an MR imaging coil: a coil with a higher filling factor produces better SNR than a coil with a lower filling factor, when other protocol parameters and patient load remain unchanged. The concept of filling factor was a first attempt to explain the inherent SNR property of a coil. It has since been replaced by a more general concept of coil sensitivity,

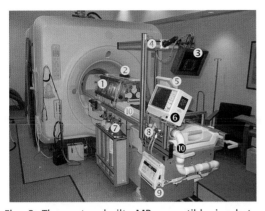

Fig. 2. The custom-built, MR-compatible incubator used at the University of California San Francisco Medical Center for neonatal MR imaging. The incubator is mounted on top of a regular MR patient table and docks to a 1.5 T SIGNA MR scanner (GE, Milwaukee, WI, USA) in the standard fashion. The design addresses the most important needs of temperature control, infant access, and monitoring of vital signs. The incubator is shown with the neonatal birdcage coil (1), infrared camera to observe the infant (2) and monitor for video display (3), equipment shelf with work lights above an integrated patient preparation table (4), an MR-compatible patient physiology monitor (Invivo, Orlando, FL, USA) (5) and remote display (6), MR-compatible air and oxygen cylinders with gas regulators (7) and gas blender (8), temperature controller and auxiliary heater box (9), and the heat transfer tube (10). (*Courtesy of* Dr C.L. Dumoulin, Cincinnati Children's Hospital.)

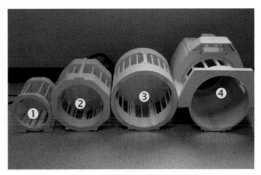

Fig. 3. Filling factor–optimized RF coils: comparison of size-optimized birdcage coils. Newborn head birdcage coil (SREE Medical Systems, Cleveland, OH, USA) optimized for MR imaging, ^{1}H MR spectroscopy (MRS), and use in the LMT MR-conditional incubator (1). SREE Medical Systems dual-tuned (^{1}H and ^{31}P) coils optimized for MR imaging and MRS in children (2) and adults (3), and General Electric standard quadrature head coil for adults (4). (*Courtesy of* Dr S. Blüml, Children's Hospital of Los Angeles.)

using the principle of reciprocity from the antenna theory.[46,50,51]

Dedicated coils tailored to the size of the neonate have been developed over the years in an attempt to bring the coil closer to the infant. **Fig. 3** shows a neonate birdcage coil for use with the LMT incubator and a size comparison with standard birdcage head coils used for adults. **Fig. 4** compares the T2-weighted images acquired with the standard birdcage (see **Fig. 3**, coil 4) and the neonate birdcage (see **Fig. 3**, coil 1) in the same infant. The higher SNR achieved with the neonate birdcage coil, approximately a factor of 3,[29] was traded for resolution and acquisition speed: the image shown in **Fig. 4**B had an 8-times higher spatial resolution and half the acquisition time compared with that shown in **Fig. 4**A.

The sensitivity of an MR imaging coil array improves not only when the array is moved closer to the patient but also when the size of the individual coil elements that form the array are optimized.[52–54] In general, coil arrays perform better if they can be adjusted in size, particularly in the anterior-posterior direction, to accommodate a larger patient population (eg, from very low birth weight premature infants to 6-month-old regular-weight infants). Another issue with adult-sized coils is that they are poorly matched to the smaller patient load when used with infants, which enhances the noise contributions from the electronics inside the coil. A dedicated pediatric coil array is better matched to neonates and therefore minimizes the image noise generated by the coil.[54]

Following these basic principles of coil design (ie, maximizing SNR by closely fitting the coils around the patient and minimizing intrinsic losses caused by coil hardware), more pediatric array coils have become available in recent years. A representative set of commercially available solutions is shown in **Fig. 5**. However, except for the integrated head-neck-spine-abdomen coil array shown in **Fig. 5**A, these coils are optimized for an older pediatric population and not for preterm and term infants, but they can still be used and offer an SNR benefit compared with adult phased array coils. In addition, they are also not compatible with the LMT incubator, which has its own current line of RF antennas with up to 12 elements. **Table 1** summarizes current commercially available pediatric coils suitable for neonate imaging.

Advanced RF Coils

A significant challenge for hardware design in MR imaging in children is the growth of patients and the large variation in patient size. As per growth charts, the average head circumference is 20 to

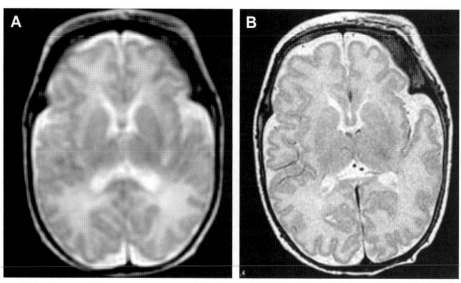

Fig. 4. T2-weighted images from a newborn obtained with the standard adult birdcage coil (*A*) and the neonate head birdcage coil integrated in the incubator (*B*). (*Courtesy of* Dr S. Blüml, Children's Hospital of Los Angeles.)

22 cm for preterm infants at 22 weeks, 38.5 cm for full-term newborns, and up to 46 cm (95 percentile) for 6-month-old babies.[55–57] A single infant head coil covering the entire size range is optimal, but the large variation in head size impedes meeting this goal. Flexible or adjustable coil arrays could be used for wider age ranges. However, there are limits in applying flexible designs to volume coils such as head coils. In addition, adjustable coils, with their more complex mechanical solutions, are not as reliable and easy to clean, the latter limitation being important in the context of very young patients. A comprehensive set of pediatric MR imaging coils should ideally contain flexible or adjustable coils for imaging of the torso/spine region, and a set of differently sized head coils.

Recent research has focused on the development of 32-channel brain arrays for pediatric neuroimaging spanning the age group of neonates to 7-year-old children (**Fig. 6**).[58] This development is a logical continuation of the success of the 32-channel brain arrays that have become standard for highest quality clinical neuroimaging in adults because of their SNR benefits[59] and ability to obtain exquisite images in reduced acquisition time by using parallel imaging techniques.[60,61] The coils shown in **Fig. 6** consist of 2 parts: a deep posterior segment laid out like a soccer ball[62] and a separate, detachable paddle with slightly larger loops that covers the forehead (**Fig. 7**).[58] The head rests deep in the posterior segment and head movement is constrained by this shape. SNR comparisons in age-matched

phantom models of the head among the set of 32-channel pediatric coils, a 32-channel adult head array, and a pediatric-sized birdcage are shown in **Fig. 8**. The SNR of the neonate 32-channel coil is 3.6 times higher at the periphery (edge of the phantom) and 1.25 times higher at the center of the phantom than that of the adult 32-channel head coil.[58] When averaged over the whole brain, the SNR of the neonate coil is still 2.8 times higher than that of the adult array. The SNR of the neonate array is 5.4 times higher at the periphery and 1.3 times higher at the center than that of the birdcage coil. The high number of coil elements combined with the high SNR significantly reduces the scanning time, which is of utmost importance in neonates. Furthermore, the likelihood of head motion is reduced during shorter scans and because of the coil design, which is an essential prerequisite for accurate functional imaging (blood oxygenation level dependent, diffusion) studies that are required during diagnostic assessment of ill preterm or term infants.

Multipurpose Infant RF Coil Design

Proper design of neonate MR imaging coils for use in an MR-conditional incubator or as a stand-alone solution requires an understanding of workflow (including transport, imaging, and monitoring). A good design of coil and equipment allows most preparation steps to be completed outside the magnet room and facilitates easy transfer of patients from the preparation station to the MR

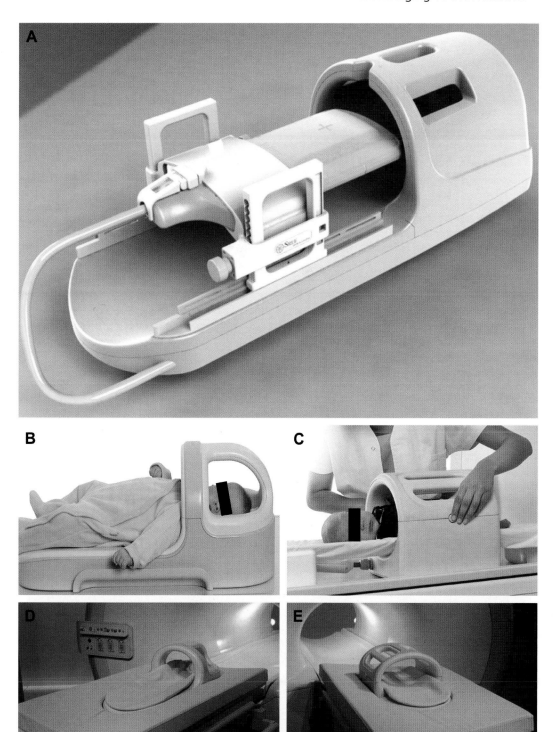

Fig. 5. Selected commercially available array coils for infants. (A) SREE Medical Systems brain/spine/cardiac array* for infants up to 6 months of age. (B) Eight-element pediatric head spine array coil (Philips, Best, Netherlands) in cradle design optimized for neonates and infants up to 10 kg. (C) Eight-element pediatric torso/cardiac array coil (Philips, Best, Netherlands) in split design for easy positioning and access to the infant. The coil covers 26 cm in the head-foot direction and is suited for high-resolution body and cardiac imaging in pediatric patients of up to 15 kg. The parallel imaging acceleration factor is 3 with coils (B) and (C). (D, E) Both coils with mattresses elevating them closer to the isocenter of the magnet, thereby possibly improving the image quality. *Pending US FDA and EU CE certification. ([A] *Courtesy of* Ravi Srinivasan, SREE Medical Systems, Cleveland, OH.)

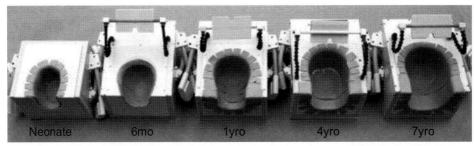

Fig. 6. Posterior coil segments of 5 constructed pediatric array coils (neonate, 6 months, 1 year, 4 years, 7 years). The coil formers are based on the 95th percentile MR imaging contours of children of the corresponding ages and have been dilated to accommodate foam padding. The coil formers were three-dimensional printed and enclosed in a plastic box. Mounted mirrors were used to project visual stimulus for research studies. (*Reprinted from* Keil B, Alagappan V, Mareyam A, et al. Size-optimized 32-channel brain arrays for 3T pediatric imaging. Magn Reson Med 2011. doi:10.1002/mrm.22961, see **Fig. 2**; with permission.)

table. Minimizing set-up time is as important as reducing scan time. Certain set-up issues can be addressed by using a dedicated coil. For example, the coil should be designed for the simultaneous use of monitoring, breathing/ventilation, and other equipment. For this reason, the coil should allow sufficient access to the infant's face to allow placement of an oxygen mask or similar equipment. A mirror should be included for easy visual observation of the patient by medical staff. Integrated cable channels and holders for monitoring equipment are an added benefit.

Precautionary measures need to be established to access the patient in emergency situations. Anterior coils have to be designed so that they can be easily removed to minimize the time to get to the neonate. Before using the equipment on a patient, all health care personnel and MR personnel involved in the scan procedure should consider practicing emergency responses by using a phantom or doll to identify potential hazards in the setup.

A head-neck-spine array with the addition of a height-adjustable anterior body array can cover most indications where MR imaging is prescribed. Small flex coils can be used in addition to this setup for increasing the SNR for some localized applications such as imaging of joints. Moving the infant closer to the magnet's isocenter can improve image quality because of higher linearity in both static magnetic field and gradients.

Dedicated neonatal coils should, like every coil, be designed to maximize the baseline SNR, which is the SNR if no parallel imaging is used. It is advantageous to use a higher coil element count combined with an element layout that allows parallel imaging (discussed later), provided it does not compromise the baseline SNR and result

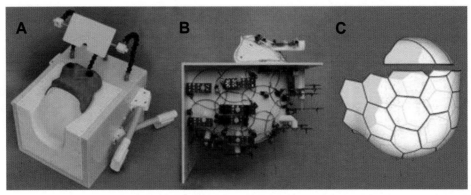

Fig. 7. The completed array coil for a 1-year-old child consists of 2 segments: a deep posterior segment and a frontal paddle over the forehead (in orange). The eyes and face of the subject are completely unobstructed. (*A*) Finalized coil enclosed in a plastic box. (*B*) Inside view of the three-dimensional printed coil formers with coil circuitry. (*C*) Tiling geometry diagram of the 32-channel layout; the loop diameters are slightly larger than the diameter of the circle that inscribes the vertexes of the hexagon/pentagons. (*Reprinted from* Keil B, Alagappan V, Mareyam A, et al. Size-optimized 32-channel brain arrays for 3T pediatric imaging. Magn Reson Med 2011. doi:10.1002/mrm.22961, see **Fig. 1**; with permission.)

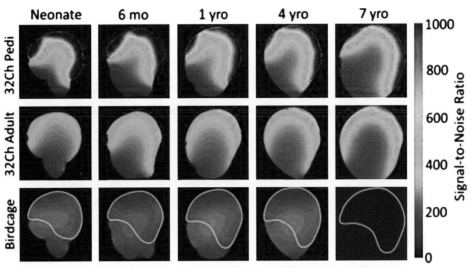

Fig. 8. SNR comparisons between sagittal images obtained from sized-matched head phantoms, using the pediatric brain array coils (*first row*), the 32-channel adult brain array coil (*second row*), and a circular polarized birdcage coil (*third row*). The images show that the highest SNR gain occurs closest to the surface of the constructed array. The SNR is only slightly improved in the brain center of the phantoms. The superimposed region of interest on the birdcage coil SNR maps correspond to the regions used in the average brain SNR measurement. The 7-year-old phantom was too big to fit into the pediatric birdcage coil. (*Reprinted from* Keil B, Alagappan V, Mareyam A, et al. Size-optimized 32-channel brain arrays for 3T pediatric imaging. Magn Reson Med 2011. doi: 10.1002/mrm. 22961, see **Fig. 5**; with permission.)

in moderate geometry factors (g-factors). Parallel imaging can reduce the scan time and help combat image artifacts and blurring caused by patient motion or relaxation decay. Use of spatial information from coil sensitivity profiles for retrospective data correction can further improve image quality.[63,64]

Fig. 9 shows a current work-in-progress head-neck-spine-body array for infants up to 18 months of age incorporating these design criteria. The array contains a total of 32 coil elements, two 3 by 3 anterior and posterior arrays covering the abdominal and spine region with a total of 18 coil elements. Another 14 elements cover the head and cervical spine region. **Fig. 9**A shows the interior of an early prototype. **Fig. 9**B shows the fully assembled prototype. The system is designed to cover the area from head to pelvis in the targeted age group.

Parallel Imaging

Imaging speed can be increased by reducing the number of averages, increasing the gradient strength, or by using improved pulse sequence techniques such as turbo spin echo (TSE), radial, spiral, or echo planar (EP) imaging. However, peripheral nerve stimulation and SAR constitute fundamental limits to the increase of imaging speed by these techniques.

Imaging speed can be further improved by using parallel imaging techniques that use coil sensitivity information to compensate for missing spatial encoding data, which otherwise have to be obtained via time-consuming additional phase-encoding steps. However, parallel imaging causes a reduction in SNR per unit time, characterized by the g-factor.[60]

When using parallel imaging, the reduced SNR (SNR_{red}) can be written as a function of the unaccelerated baseline SNR (SNR_{full}), the speed-up or reduction factor R, and the coil-specific and patient-specific geometry factor g:

$$SNR_{red} = \frac{SNR_{full}}{g\sqrt{R}}$$

Note that g is greater than or equal to 1, and therefore the minimum penalty in SNR is for g = 1 or at least the square root of the acceleration factor R. Without the g-factor, the SNR is proportional to the square root of the total scan time, which means that cutting scan time in half reduces SNR by the square root of 2 or roughly 30%.

Coil arrays designed for parallel imaging combat the g-factor by optimizing the coil element layout and increasing the total number of coil channels. In general, increasing the number of coil elements along the phase-encoding direction improves spatial information and thereby reduces the g-factor. The rule of thumb is that the number of

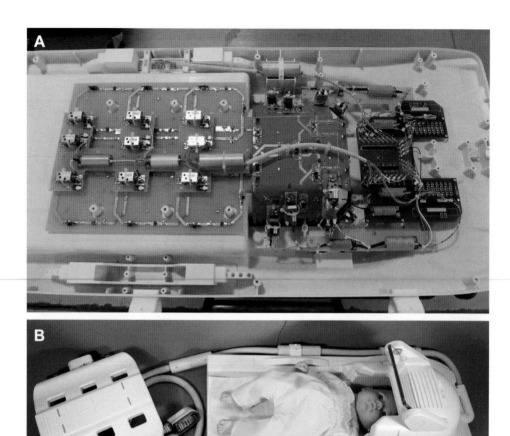

Fig. 9. Prototype of a 32-channel pediatric coil array for head, neck, spine, and body imaging (Invivo, Orlando, FL, USA). The array contains a total of 32 coil elements: a 3 × 3 anterior and a 3 × 3 posterior coil array cover the abdominal and spine region with a total of 18 coils; another 14 elements cover the head and cervical spine region. The arrays are designed to cover the area from head to pelvis in infants up to 18 months of age. (*A*) The interior of a prototype, and (*B*) fully assembled prototype.

coil elements in the phase-encoding direction should be higher than the scan time reduction factor. However, the g-factor is not a constant and increases with the reduction factor. For high reduction factors, even an ideal coil array with a coil element count approaching infinity has a limiting g-factor higher than 1, called the ultimate g-factor.[65–68] Also, increasing the number of coil elements while decreasing the individual element size can introduce additional losses and reduce the baseline SNR.[69]

DEDICATED NICU SCANNERS

When MR imaging is clinically indicated in critically ill preterm or term infants, they should ideally be examined in the NICU itself, thereby avoiding transportation to the radiology department. Dedicated NICU scanners not only obviate transporting the patient but also allow a more flexible schedule of imaging that can better accommodate the sleeping patterns and needs of the infant.

However, to our knowledge there are currently only 2 functional MR installations in the NICU worldwide: a standard 3 T MR imaging scanner (upgrade from a prior customized 1 T system)[70] at Hammersmith Hospital, London, United Kingdom, and a 0.17 T specialized MR scanner at Jessop Hospital, Sheffield, United Kingdom.[71] A third system based on an orthopedic 1.5 T scanner is currently being developed at Cincinnati Children's Hospital, Ohio.[72] The upgrade from a 1 T to 3 T at Hammersmith attests that neonatal examinations, especially structural imaging, functional imaging, and spectroscopy, can benefit from the threefold higher SNR or the improved spatial and temporal resolution obtained at a higher magnetic field strength. Although commercial high-field scanners with their wide range of MR sequences are ideal for neonatal MR imaging, their widespread use in NICUs may be hindered by practical issues (apart from cost) such as (1) weight of the magnets (5–6 tons for modern 1.5-T and 3-T systems), which may not be supported by most existing building structures that house the NICU; (2) space requirements; and (3) the large three-dimensional fringe field that may interfere with not only NICU life support and monitoring equipment but also with other medical equipment in floors above and below the NICU.

Researchers at Cincinnati Children's Hospital bypassed these limitations by developing a customized MR scanner designed specifically for neonates and for installation in the NICU.[72] Unlike the whole-body system used at Hammersmith, a small, 1.5-T MR system (Optima MR430s 1.5T, GE Healthcare, Waukesha, WI) designed for adult orthopedic applications has been adapted for neonatal use at Cincinnati Children's Hospital (**Fig. 10**). The magnet weighs only 408 kg. The

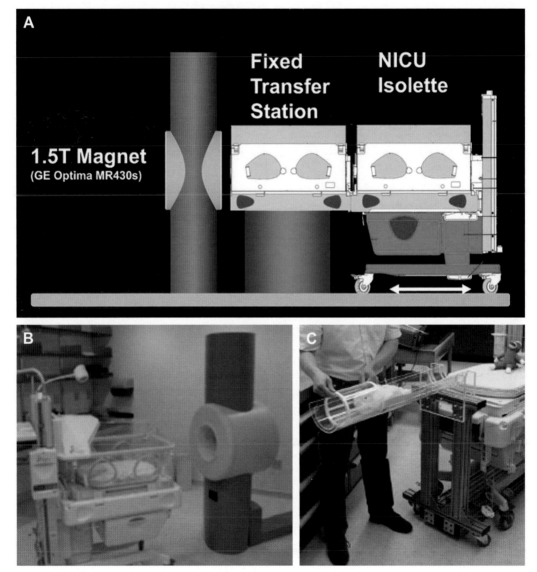

Fig. 10. Development of a dedicated NICU MR system at Cincinnati Children's Medical Center (CCHMC). (*A*) The design concept. (*B*) The prototype installation with incubator in a biosafety level 2 laboratory of the Imaging Research Center at CCHMC, and (*C*) the baby holder/cradle and a mock-up of a birdcage head coil. (*Courtesy of* Drs C.L. Dumoulin and J.A. Tkach, Cincinnati Children's Hospital.)

scanner has a patient bore of diameter 21.8 cm, and has a gradient strength of 70 mT/m and slew rate of 300 T/m/s, almost twice that of high-end whole-body systems. These parameters are obtainable in the Optima MR430s 1.5T because of the small geometric size of the gradients, which facilitates fast imaging (optimized EP imaging sequences for perfusion and functional imaging studies with reduced motion artifacts) and advanced diffusion imaging and tractography by using high b-values, without triggering peripheral nerve stimulation. Small gradients also reduce

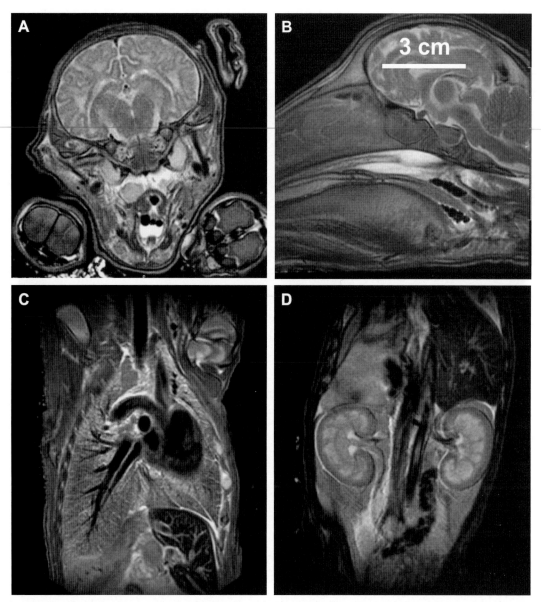

Fig. 11. Representative images obtained in newborn lambs, using the Cincinnati NICU MR imaging prototype system. High-quality T2-weighted TSE images of the brain (*A*, *B*). The voxel size in each is 0.35 × 0.35 × 2 mm^3, with acquisition parameters TR = 3000 ms, TE = 120 ms, field of view (FOV) = 90 mm, matrix = 256 × 256, slice thickness = 2 mm, echo train length (ETL) = 12, receiver bandwidth (BW) = 50 kHz, 5 acquisitions; scan time = 5:20 min. Other applications include lung (*C*) and kidneys (*D*). Acquisition parameters for (*C*) and (*D*) were TSE, TR = 3000 ms, TE = 81 ms, FOV = 145 mm, matrix = 256 × 256, slice thickness = 3 mm, voxel size = 0.57 × 0.57 × 3 mm^3, ETL = 8, receiver BW = 50 kHz, 4 acquisitions, scan time = 6:24 min. (*Courtesy of* Drs C.L. Dumoulin and J.A. Tkach, Cincinnati Children's Hospital.)

the acoustic noise. Researchers at Cincinnati Children's Hospital are also developing an MR-compatible incubator and transfer station. The transfer station enables continuous temperature regulation and physiologic monitoring to be maintained throughout the MR imaging examination without untethering the baby from the incubator. The last step is to integrate the system with a standard GE console to allow full access to state-of-the-art imaging (eg, spiral, propeller, parallel and diffusion tensor imaging, and spectroscopy), ECG triggering, and respiratory capabilities, in addition to sequence programming. **Fig. 11** shows the first images obtained with this system: preterm twin sheep were delivered by cesarean section at approximately 85% of their full gestational age. These lambs were roughly the same size, shape, and weight as the human neonate, making them a good model to study premature birth. A 14.5-cm volume coil was used to acquire images during the first few hours of life. Ventilation, temperature regulation, and physiologic monitoring were maintained during the examination by using the same strategies and equipment as required for scanning human neonates. Standard SE, TSE, and GE sequences were used to acquire images of the brain, spine, chest, and abdomen. ECG and respiratory gating/triggering were not available at the time of these experiments. T2 images of the brain show high spatial resolution and good tissue contrast (see **Fig. 11**A, B), and the images of the chest and abdomen are free of artifacts (see **Fig. 11**C, D), even without respiratory and ECG gating,[72] rendering this NICU system a promising prototype.

SUMMARY

This article describes the requirements, challenges, practical issues, complexities, and risks associated with neonatal MR imaging and reviews available equipment and common procedures for MR-related transport, sedation, monitoring, and scanning of neonates. MR plays an increasingly important role in the diagnosis and clinical management of critically ill, very low birth weight preterm or full-term infants, so active research is ongoing to make the transport and examination safer and imaging more successful (ie, shorter and free of motion artifacts). Efforts are focused on (1) integration of dedicated neonate MR scanners in the NICU; (2) improvements in incubator technology and handling; (3) more efficient use of the scan/sedation time by choosing dedicated neonate coil arrays that improve the SNR and facilitate the choice of modern imaging techniques, such as parallel imaging.

ACKNOWLEDGMENTS

The authors thank Drs Jean Tkach and Charles Demoulin from Cincinnati Children's Hospital and Dr Stefan Blüml from the Children's Hospital Los Angeles for providing information and figures. The authors thank Ms Molly Rollen and Dr Ralf Loeffler from St Jude Children's Research Hospital in Memphis for support and helpful discussions and Dr Vani Shanker, also from St. Jude, for scientific editing of the article.

REFERENCES

1. Mathur AM, Neil JJ, McKinstry RC, et al. Transport, monitoring, and successful brain MR imaging in unsedated neonates. Pediatr Radiol 2008;38(3):260–4.
2. van Wezel-Meijler G, Leijser LM, de Bruine FT, et al. Magnetic resonance imaging of the brain in newborn infants: practical aspects. Early Hum Dev 2009;85(2):85–92.
3. Counsell SJ, Rutherford MA, Cowan FM, et al. Magnetic resonance imaging of preterm brain injury. Arch Dis Child Fetal Neonatal Ed 2003;88(4): F269–74.
4. Rona Z, Klebermass K, Cardona F, et al. Comparison of neonatal MRI examinations with and without an MR-compatible incubator: advantages in examination feasibility and clinical decision-making. Eur J Paediatr Neurol 2010;14(5):410–7.
5. Woodward LJ, Anderson PJ, Austin NC, et al. Neonatal MRI to predict neurodevelopmental outcomes in preterm infants. N Engl J Med 2006; 355(7):685–94.
6. Ment LR, Bada HS, Barnes P, et al. Practice parameter: neuroimaging of the neonate: report of the Quality Standards Subcommittee of the American Academy of Neurology and the Practice Committee of the Child Neurology Society. Neurology 2002; 58(12):1726–38.
7. O'Shea TM, Counsell SJ, Bartels DB, et al. Magnetic resonance and ultrasound brain imaging in preterm infants. Early Hum Dev 2005;81(3):263–71.
8. Leijser LM, Liauw L, Veen S, et al. Comparing brain white matter on sequential cranial ultrasound and MRI in very preterm infants. Neuroradiology 2008; 50(9):799–811.
9. Panigrahy A, Bluml S. Advances in magnetic resonance neuroimaging techniques in the evaluation of neonatal encephalopathy. Top Magn Reson Imaging 2007;18(1):3–29.
10. Panigrahy A, Borzage M, Bluml S. Basic principles and concepts underlying recent advances in magnetic resonance imaging of the developing brain. Semin Perinatol 2010;34(1):3–19.
11. Wilder RT, Flick RP, Sprung J, et al. Early exposure to anesthesia and learning disabilities in a

population-based birth cohort. Anesthesiology 2009;110(4):796–804.

12. Rutherford M, Srinivasan L, Dyet L, et al. Magnetic resonance imaging in perinatal brain injury: clinical presentation, lesions and outcome. Pediatr Radiol 2006;36(7):582–92.

13. Kanal E, Barkovich AJ, Bell C, et al. ACR guidance document for safe MR practices: 2007. AJR Am J Roentgenol 2007;188(6):1447–74.

14. Stokowski LA. Ensuring safety for infants undergoing magnetic resonance imaging. Adv Neonatal Care 2005;5(1):14–27 [quiz: 52–14].

15. Benavente-Fernandez I, Lubian-Lopez PS, Zuazo-Ojeda MA, et al. Safety of magnetic resonance imaging in preterm infants. Acta Paediatr 2010; 99(6):850–3.

16. Pennock JM. Patient preparation, safety and hazards in imaging infants and children. In: Rutherford MA, editor. MRI of the neonatal brain. Saunders Ltd; 2001. Chapter 01. Available at: http://www.mrineonatalbrain.com. Accessed March 14, 2011.

17. Woods TO. Guidance for industry and FDA staff: establishing safety and compatibility of passive implants in the magnetic resonance (MR) environment. Rockville (MD): Food and Drug Administration; 2008.

18. ASTM. Standard practice for marking medical devices and other items for safety in the magnetic resonance environment. Vol F2503-05. West Conshohocken (PA): ASTM International; 2005.

19. Reykowski A. RF coil safety - weekend categorical course. Joint Annual Meeting ISMRM-ESMRMB. Berlin (Germany), May 19–25, 2007.

20. EN/IEC 60601-2-33-Medical Electrical Equipment - Part 2: particular requirements for the safety of magnetic resonance equipment for medical diagnosis. IEC 60601: International Standard.

21. Guidance for industry and FDA staff. Criteria for significant risk investigations of magnetic resonance diagnostic devices. Rockville (MD): Food and Drug Administration; 2003.

22. Maalouf EF, Counsell SJ. Imaging the preterm infant: practical issues. In: Rutherford MA, editor. MRI of the neonatal brain. Saunders Ltd; 2001. Chapter 02. Available at: http://www.mrineonatalbrain.com. Accessed March 14, 2011.

23. Murkovic I, Steinberg MD, Murkovic B. Sensors in neonatal monitoring: current practice and future trends. Technol Health Care 2003;11(6):399–412.

24. Theobald K, Botwinski C, Albanna S, et al. Apnea of prematurity: diagnosis, implications for care, and pharmacologic management. Neonatal Netw 2000; 19(6):17–24.

25. Philbin MK, Taber KH, Hayman LA. Preliminary report: changes in vital signs of term newborns during MR. AJNR Am J Neuroradiol 1996;17(6): 1033–6.

26. Taber KH, Hayman LA, Northrup SR, et al. Vital sign changes during infant magnetic resonance examinations. J Magn Reson Imaging 1998;8(6):1252–6.

27. Shellock FG. Reference manual for magnetic resonance safety, implants, and devices: 2011 edition. Los Angeles (CA): Biomedical Research Publishing Group; 2011.

28. LMT Lammers Medical Technology GmbH. MR diagnostics incubator system nomag® IC installed units. 2011. Available at: http://lammersmedical.com/e/pages/about-us/customer.php. Accessed September 24, 2011.

29. Bluml S, Friedlich P, Erberich S, et al. MR imaging of newborns by using an MR-compatible incubator with integrated radiofrequency coils: initial experience. Radiology 2004;231(2):594–601.

30. Erberich SG, Friedlich P, Seri I, et al. Functional MRI in neonates using neonatal head coil and MR compatible incubator. Neuroimage 2003;20(2): 683–92.

31. Whitby EH, Griffiths PD, Lonneker-Lammers T, et al. Ultrafast magnetic resonance imaging of the neonate in a magnetic resonance-compatible incubator with a built-in coil. Pediatrics 2004;113(2): e150–2.

32. Dumoulin CL, Rohling KW, Piel JE, et al. Magnetic resonance imaging compatible neonate incubator. Concept Magnetic Res 2002;15(2):117–28.

33. Barkovich AJ. MR imaging of the neonatal brain. Neuroimaging Clin N Am 2006;16(1):117–35, viii-ix.

34. Prager A, Roychowdhury S. Magnetic resonance imaging of the neonatal brain. Indian J Pediatr 2007;74(2):173–84.

35. Greenberg SB, Faerber EN, Aspinall CL, et al. High-dose chloral hydrate sedation for children undergoing MR imaging: safety and efficacy in relation to age. AJR Am J Roentgenol 1993;161(3):639–41.

36. Bisset GS 3rd, Ball WS Jr. Preparation, sedation, and monitoring of the pediatric patient in the magnetic resonance suite. Semin Ultrasound CT MR 1991;12(5):376–8.

37. Rutherford M, Malamateniou C, McGuinness A, et al. Magnetic resonance imaging in hypoxic-ischaemic encephalopathy. Early Human Dev 2010;86(6): 351–60.

38. Litman RS, Soin K, Salam A. Chloral hydrate sedation in term and preterm infants: an analysis of efficacy and complications. Anesth Analg 2010; 110(3):739–46.

39. Rutherford MA, Ward P, Malamatentiou C. Advanced MR techniques in the term-born neonate with perinatal brain injury. Semin Fetal Neonatal Med 2005; 10(5):445–60.

40. Mason KP. The pediatric sedation service: who is appropriate to sedate, which medications should I use, who should prescribe the drugs, how do I bill? Pediatr Radiol 2008;38(Suppl 2):S218–24.

41. Shankar VR. Sedating children for radiological procedures: an intensivist's perspective. Pediatr Radiol 2008;38(Suppl 2):S213–7.

42. Mellon RD, Simone AF, Rappaport BA. Use of anesthetic agents in neonates and young children. Anesth Analg 2007;104(3):509–20.

43. Vigneron DB, Barkovich AJ, Noworolski SM, et al. Three-dimensional proton MR spectroscopic imaging of premature and term neonates. AJNR Am J Neuroradiol 2001;22(7):1424–33.

44. Dagia C, Ditchfield M. 3T MRI in paediatrics: challenges and clinical applications. Eur J Radiol 2008; 68(2):309–19.

45. Kliegman MR, Behrman RE, Jenson HB, et al. Nelson textbook of pediatrics e-dition, 18th edition & atlas of pediatric physical diagnosis, 5th edition package. 18th edition. Philadelphia: Saunders; 2007.

46. Hoult D, Richards R. The signal-to-noise ratio of the nuclear magnetic resonance experiment. JMR 1976; 24:71–85.

47. Edelstein WA, Glover GH, Hardy CJ, et al. The intrinsic signal-to-noise ratio in NMR imaging. Magn Reson Med 1986;3(4):604–18.

48. Arthur R. Magnetic resonance imaging in preterm infants. Pediatr Radiol 2006;36(7):593–607.

49. Abragam A. The principles of nuclear magnetism. 3rd edition. Oxford (United Kingdom): Clarendon Press; 1983.

50. Harrington R. Time-harmonic electromagnetic fields. New York: McGraw-Hill; 1961.

51. Vesselle H. High-frequency electromagnetic effects and signal-to-noise ratios of surface coils for magnetic resonance imaging [PhD dissertation]. Cleveland (OH): Case Western Reserve University; 1990.

52. Wang J, Reykowski A, Dickas J. Calculation of the signal-to-noise ratio for simple surface coils and arrays of coils. IEEE Trans Biomed Eng 1995;42(9): 908–17.

53. Roemer P, Edelstein WA. Ultimate sensitivity limit of surface coils. SMRM 6th Annual Meeting. New York (NY), 1987. p. 410.

54. Schnell W, Renz W, Vester M, et al. Ultimate signal-to-noise-ratio of surface and body antennas for magnetic resonance imaging. IEEE T Antenn Propag 2000;48(3):418–28.

55. Ehrenkranz RA, Younes N, Lemons JA, et al. Longitudinal growth of hospitalized very low birth weight infants. Pediatrics 1999;104(2 Pt 1):280–9.

56. Kuczmarski RJ, Ogden CL, Grummer-Strawn LM, et al. CDC growth charts: United States. Adv Data 2000;(314):1–27.

57. Fenton TR. A new growth chart for preterm babies: Babson and Benda's chart updated with recent data and a new format. BMC Pediatr 2003;3:13.

58. Keil B, Alagappan V, Mareyam A, et al. Size-optimized 32-channel brain arrays for 3 T pediatric imaging. Magn Reson Med 2011. DOI:10.1002/mrm.22961. [Epub ahead of print].

59. Parikh PT, Sandhu GS, Blackham KA, et al. Evaluation of image quality of a 32-channel versus a 12-channel head coil at 1.5T for MR imaging of the brain. AJNR Am J Neuroradiol 2011;32(2): 365–73.

60. Pruessmann KP, Weiger M, Scheidegger MB, et al. Sensitivity encoding for fast MRI. Magn Reson Med 1999;42(5):952–62.

61. Griswold MA, Jakob PM, Heidemann RM, et al. Generalized autocalibrating partially parallel acquisitions (GRAPPA). Magn Reson Med 2002;47(6): 1202–10.

62. Wiggins GC, Triantafyllou C, Potthast A, et al. 32-channel 3 Tesla receive-only phased-array head coil with soccer-ball element geometry. Magn Reson Med 2006;56(1):216–23.

63. Horbar JD, Badger GJ, Carpenter JH, et al. Trends in mortality and morbidity for very low birth weight infants, 1991-1999. Pediatrics 2002;110(1 Pt 1): 143–51.

64. Lin W, Huang F, Bornert P, et al. Motion correction using an enhanced floating navigator and GRAPPA operations. Magn Reson Med 2010; 63(2):339–48.

65. Reykowski A, Schnell W, Wang J. Simulation of SNR limit for SENSE related reconstruction techniques [abstract]. Honolulu (HI): ISMRM; 2002. p. 2385.

66. Reykowski A. How to calculate the SNR limit of SENSE related reconstruction techniques [abstract]. Honolulu (HI): ISMRM; 2002. p. 905.

67. Ohliger MA, Grant AK, Sodickson DK. Ultimate intrinsic signal-to-noise ratio for parallel MRI: electromagnetic field considerations. Magn Reson Med 2003;50(5):1018–30.

68. Wiesinger F, Boesiger P, Pruessmann KP. Electrodynamics and ultimate SNR in parallel MR imaging. Magn Reson Med 2004;52(2):376–90.

69. Duensing GR, Akao J, Saylor C, et al. Conductor losses in many channel RF coil arrays. Kyoto (Japan): ISMRM; 2004. p. 1583.

70. Hall AS, Young IR, Davies FJ, et al. A dedicated magnetic resonance system in a neonatal intensive therapy unit. In: Bradley WG, Bydder GM, editors. Advanced MR imaging techniques. London: Martin Dunitz; 1997. p. 281–9.

71. Whitby EH, Paley MN, Smith MF, et al. Low field strength magnetic resonance imaging of the neonatal brain. Arch Dis Child Fetal Neonatal Ed 2003;88(3):F203–8.

72. Tkach JA, Giaquinto R, Loew W, et al. Imaging system for imaging neonates in the NICU. Paper presented at: 6th Congress and Exhibition of the Joint Societies of Paediatric Radiology. London, May 29, 2011.

Advanced Neonatal NeuroMRI

Kenichi Oishi, MD, PhD[a],*, Andreia V. Faria, MD, PhD[a],
Susumu Mori, PhD[a,b]

KEYWORDS

- Neonate • Diffusion tensor imaging • Normalization
- Quantification • Brain atlas

Recent advances in MR imaging techniques enable scanning of the neonatal brain with various techniques. These include structural MR imaging (T1- and T2-weighted images), diffusion tensor imaging (DTI), perfusion MR imaging, functional MR imaging, MR angiography, and MR spectroscopy. However, because of the small size of the neonate brain, limited scan time, and image contrasts that are very different from adult brains, there are unique issues that must be addressed to develop an effective quantitative neonate MR imaging technique. This article focuses on a state-of-the-art quantification method for structural MR imaging and DTI of neonates, which helps to deepen the understanding of human brain development, and the potential for the clinical application of quantitative MR imaging techniques.

IMPORTANCE OF NEONATAL BRAIN MR IMAGING ANALYSIS

The brain suffers various insults during the prenatal and perinatal period, such as hypoxia–ischemia, infection, and exposure to toxic substances. There are also genetic abnormalities that affect brain development. Preterm birth and low birth weight are also risk factors for brain damage. Severely damaged babies show abnormal symptoms immediately after birth. Mild to moderate damage has been linked to abnormalities later in life. For example, approximately 50% of babies born at very preterm, defined as less than or equal to 32 gestational weeks, are at risk for developing cerebral palsy, epilepsy, impaired academic achievement, and behavioral disorders, including attention-deficit/hyperactivity disorder.[1–3] However, most neuropsychologic impairments are not obvious during the first year of life. Therefore, a symptom-based diagnosis is extremely difficult for neonates with mild to moderate brain damage. For successful early interventions, an effective evaluation method is needed to detect and characterize brain damage as early as possible. Evaluation of neonatal brain damage using MR imaging has several advantages. First, MR imaging is sensitive for the detection of subtle brain abnormalities compared with other imaging modalities, such as CT and ultrasound. Previous studies using conventional T1- and T2-weighted images indicate that an expert radiologist can detect some abnormality in 70% of MR scans from very preterm infants.[4] Second, the scanning of nonsedated neonates is better for the neonate, and progressively becomes more difficult until the fourth year of life, because of the greater motion and shorter sleep time. Neonates can be scanned during hospitalization, which is another advantage. In addition, MR imaging is now widely available and, once the protocol and image-processing stream are accomplished, they can be performed and implemented on routine clinical scanners.

This work was supported by Grant No. R21AG033774 and R01HD065955 from the National Institutes of Health.
a The Russell H. Morgan Department of Radiology and Radiological Science, The Johns Hopkins University School of Medicine, 217 Traylor Building, 720 Rutland Avenue, Baltimore, MD 21205, USA
b F.M. Kirby Research Center for Functional Brain Imaging, Kennedy Krieger Institute, 707 North Broadway, Baltimore, MD 21205, USA
* Corresponding author.
E-mail address: koishi@mri.jhu.edu

mri.theclinics.com

FEATURES OF THE NEONATAL BRAIN MR IMAGING

Anatomy of the Neonatal Brain

The most striking difference between the neonatal brain and the adult brain is size. The neonatal brain volume is approximately one-third to one-fourth that of the adult brain. Inside the brain, the immature architecture is constantly developing. The cerebral cortex develops sequentially. The most prominent neuronal form in the neonatal brain is the pyramidal cell. Pyramidal cells are guided from the deep part of the brain (subventricular zone) to the cortical area (the subplate, a transient developmental layer of the cortex) during 12 to 20 weeks gestation. After they arrive at the subplate, pyramidal neurons begin to make synapses and elaborate a dendritic tree. The axons and dendrites, along with fine glial processes, make up the neuropil. At term, pyramidal cells dominate the cortex, but the neuropil development is still insufficient. Pyramidal cells have a prominent apical dendrite extending from the top of the cell body to layer I; these large dendrites give a strong radial orientation to the cortex.

Myelination of the human brain begins at approximately 29 weeks of gestation in the telencephalon.[5] The myelin sheath is formed by oligodendrocytes. The oligodendrocyte and its product, myelin, are synergistic with the developing axon[6] (ie, the axonal cytoskeleton does not form properly in the absence of myelin),[7] whereas the amount of myelin formed by the oligodendrocyte is controlled by the rate of expansion of the growing axonal cylinder.[8] Myelination proceeds in a temporally and spatially inhomogeneous manner.[6] Specifically, tracts in the brain myelinate at different rates and times. At term, the axonal network is still developing and the myelination is insufficient in most of the white matter structures, except for some tracts in the brainstem.

Structural MR Imaging of the Neonatal Brain

The neonatal brain is immature. On T1-weighted images, the intensity of the white matter is lower than that of the gray matter. On T2-weighted images, the intensity of the white matter is higher than that of the gray matter. These contrasts are the reverse of those seen in adults (**Fig. 1**). This is caused by incomplete myelination in the white matter of the neonatal brain. Because of the variability of myelination status in different fibers, the contrast between the gray and white matter in some areas is very poor. For example, the anterior limb of the internal capsule is one of the most myelinated areas at term. Consequently, the signal intensity of this structure on T2-weighted images is lower than the other white matter areas and very close to that of the surrounding gray matter structures. Although identification of this area is easy on T2-weighted images in the adult, it is extremely difficult in the neonatal brain (**Fig. 2**). To quantify the absolute T1 and T2 relaxation time of each brain structure, a quantitative T1 map and T2 maps can be created, in which T1 and T2 relaxation time are measured at each pixel. For example, the T2 map, which is often used to evaluate the myelination status of the brain, can be calculated from dual or multiple echo fast spin echo sequences by fitting the images with different echo times to an exponential model.

From MR imaging studies of normal postnatal brain development, several important time-dependent MR imaging signal changes, such as a shortening of T1 and T2 relaxation times of the gray and white matter,[9–12] have been described previously. Most of the time-dependent changes are attributed to an increase in lipid concentration caused by the myelination process.[13–17] Because the white matter appears as hyperintense on newborn T2-weighted images, the rapid shortening of T2 in the white matter results in "contrast inversion" between the white and gray matter during postnatal development (**Fig. 3**).

DTI OF THE NEONATAL BRAIN

DTI is a technique that can provide unique image contrasts inside the brain.[18–21] MR imaging can measure the extent of water diffusion (ie, the random motion of water) along an arbitrary axis. From this measurement, it is often found that water tends to diffuse along a preferential axis, which has been shown to coincide with the orientation of ordered structures, such as fiber tracts. Based on the diffusion orientation of water molecules, this technique can provide several types of new imaging contrasts, such as anisotropy maps and orientation maps, or a combination of the two, which is called a "color-coded orientation map" or simply a "color map" (**Fig. 4**). One of the most widely used metrics of diffusion anisotropy is fractional anisotropy (FA),[21,22] in which anisotropy is scaled from 0 (isotropic) to 1 (anisotropic). In the color map, the brightness shows the extent of the anisotropy and the color represents fiber orientation (see **Fig. 4**).

DTI can reveal the detailed white matter anatomy of premyelinated brains. In **Fig. 2**, white matter tracts (indicated by white labels) can be clearly identified on the color map, but not on the T2-weighted images of the neonatal brain at 40 postconception weeks. This suggests that the diffusion measurement is sensitive to axonal geometry rather than myelination. It is thus likely that the

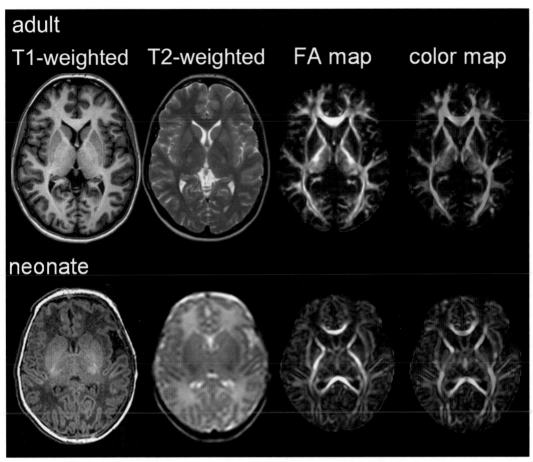

Fig. 1. Comparison between adult and neonate MR imaging. The white matter/gray matter contrast of the neonatal brain is inverted in T1- and T2-weighted images. The white matter structures of the neonate show a lower fractional anisotropy (FA) than the adult. However, the cortex has a higher FA.

anisotropy measurements allow the monitoring of axonal injuries. During the postnatal period, the anisotropy of the white matter further increases (see Fig. 3).[13,15,20,23–25] This is likely caused by myelination of the axons, although it could also be caused by an increase in axonal density or axon caliber. The diffusion anisotropy of the neonatal cortex is higher than that of adults, because of neatly aligned large dendrites of the pyramidal cells in the cortex. Anisotropy of the cortex decreases rapidly after birth, suggesting that the development of dendritic arbors in the neuropil[15,20,24] destroys the coherent water motion along the columnar organization of the cortex.

COMPLEMENTARY ROLE OF STRUCTURAL MR IMAGING AND DTI

Structural MR imaging and DTI are complementary techniques. DTI provides superior anatomic information about premyelinated brains, but less information about myelination status

compared with a T2 map. Indeed, myelination increases the anisotropy of water molecules, but other factors, such as axon and neuropil development, also affect anisotropy, which makes it less specific as an indicator of myelination. One of the biggest problems with T2 maps is, ironically, their high sensitivity to the myelination process. A T2 map is a very poor tool with which to describe the anatomy of premyelinated brains. Especially during the contrast inversion period, T2 maps often cannot even differentiate the gray and white matter. Unless one can discretely identify anatomic units of interest, one cannot quantify their T2 values in an anatomy-specific manner.

CURRENT CLINICAL APPLICATIONS FOR NEONATAL BRAIN MR IMAGING

Conventional T1- and T2-weighted images already have the ability to detect brain malformations, intracranial hemorrhage, ischemic–hypoxic injury,

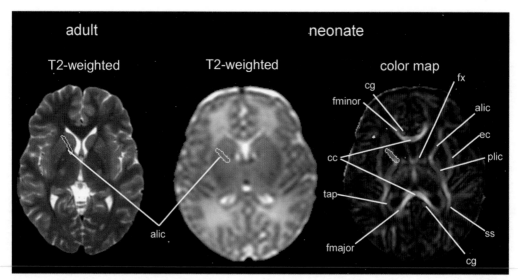

Fig. 2. An example of an adult T2-weighted image and a neonatal T2-weighted image and color map. The anterior limb of the internal capsule is identified in the adult T2-weighted image, but difficult to identify in the neonatal T2-weighted image. Using a color map, various white matter structures can be readily identified, even in the poorly myelinated neonatal brain. Coordinates of the anterior limb of the internal capsule were transferred from the color map to the T2-weighted image. alic/plic, anterior and posterior limb of internal capsule; cc, corpus callosum; cg, cingulum; ec, external capsule; fmajor/fminor, forceps major and minor; fx, fornix; ss, sagittal striatum; tap, tapatum.

signal alteration of the gray and white matter caused by seizure or metabolic abnormalities, atrophy, and ventricular enlargement. Some of these imaging features can be related to the prognosis. In the white matter area, periventricular hemorrhagic infarction and cystic periventricular white matter damage are associated with poor motor outcome,[26,27] and thinning of the corpus callosum is related to cerebral palsy and motor delay.[28] Gray matter loss and ventricular enlargement have been correlated with neurologic outcome at 1 year.[29] However, there have been studies that indicate that diffuse periventricular leukomalacia, ventricular size, and the surface area of the corpus callosum do not correlate with neurologic outcomes. The problem is that each

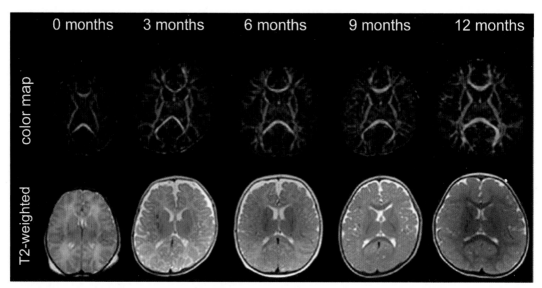

Fig. 3. Color map and T2-weighted images of 0- to 12-month-old infants. (*From* Susumu M. Introduction to diffusion tensor imaging. Amsterdam (The Netherlands): Elsevier; 2007. p. 159; with permission.)

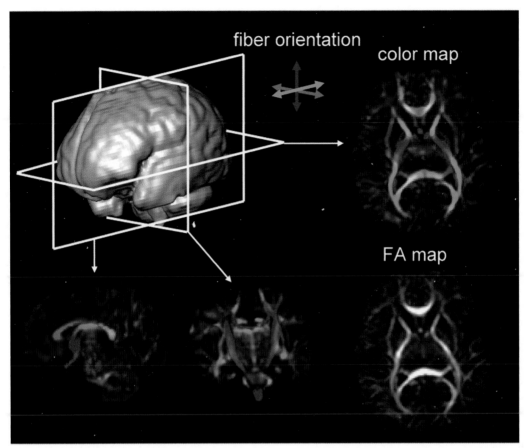

Fig. 4. DTI-based images of a neonatal brain. The raw data are three-dimensional and arbitrary slice angles and positions can be extracted. The FA and color maps have the same image intensity, but the color map has additional orientation information represented by colors. In the color map, fibers orienting along the right-left, dorsal-ventral, and caudal-rostral axes are indicated by the red, blue, and green colors, respectively.

study has used different measurements to evaluate imaging features and clinical outcomes, which makes it difficult to compare these results. Therefore, the neurologic prognostic capability is still controversial.

FROM QUALITATIVE TO QUANTITATIVE ANALYSIS

Requirements for Data Quantification

Although conventional T1- and T2-weighted images have been valuable tools to diagnose gross brain injuries, more subtle or diffuse damage has often been difficult to study. To improve the accuracy of abnormality detection and to extract more objective findings, a quantitative evaluation is required. If one can provide quantitative measures, such as volumes, shapes, and various MR parameters (eg, T1, T2, anisotropy, diffusivity) of various brain regions of the patient, and the normal range and cut-off values, one can use those measures

much like the results of blood tests are used. This not only would draw attention to potentially abnormal areas, but also provide new ways to evaluate MR images, thus expanding the ability of MR-based diagnosis by enabling one to detect previously hard-to-define abnormalities. The numbers would enable a clinician to conduct a statistical comparison between diagnostic groups, and also provide the potential to estimate the impact on the neurologic symptom or future neurologic outcomes, which is important for neonatal brain studies. Such research will be an important foundation to create diagnostic guidelines. Toward this end, there is a need to establish a data quantification method as an initial step.

Strategy for Data Quantification

For data quantification, areas from which to extract the MR parameters need to be defined (eg, T2 values). The defined area is often called a region of interest (ROI). There are three axes to define the ROI: size (large or small); number (single or multiple); and the way the area is defined (manual or automated). For example, the manual ROI method is a straightforward approach to measure MR parameters of the specific brain structure with rich localized information. However, the number of ROIs is usually limited because drawing an ROI is labor-intensive and time-consuming. This causes insufficient spatial specificity of the findings because huge brain areas remain unsurveyed. The ROIs are placed according to the a priori hypothesis, which means that this type of analysis can only be applicable for hypothesis-driven studies. There is also an issue with reproducibility. For the ROI drawing, corresponding image slice levels and locations of the brain structures among different subjects are judged based on anatomic features. However, adjusting brain position and angle at the time of the scan is not easy in the neonate brain. The ROI drawing itself requires anatomic knowledge about the neonatal brain; therefore, the reproducibility depends on the operator's skill. To achieve high reproducibility, one can increase the size of the ROI. In an extreme case, one can identify the entire brain as an ROI. In this case, one can define the ROI within a subject or across subjects with almost perfect reproducibility, but there is no localized information. In general, a manual ROI method has the inverse relationship between reproducibility and spatial information. Therefore, the other end of the extreme is using a voxel as the ROI, which has the most localization information. However, matching voxel-to-voxel manually across subjects is almost impossible.

For the initial step toward clinical application, it is necessary to screen a whole brain with rich spatial information. To handle large amounts of image data, an automated method is preferable. Voxel-based analyses, which perform the automated whole-brain voxel matching using computer software, seemed suitable for this purpose. Matching all voxels to corresponding voxels between two brains means transforming the shape of one to the other. This procedure is often called "normalization." It has the highest possible localized information. The reproducibility depends on the method used for the image normalization, which is discussed later.

Statistical analysis after normalization of an individual brain to an atlas space is an effective quantification strategy to detect differences between a target group and a control group without an a priori hypothesis. This strategy is also suitable for automated detection of the pathology. One important drawback of this voxel-based statistical comparison is the low sensitivity for detecting wide-spread subtle abnormalities. Because of the large number of the voxels and the noise, it is not easy to achieve statistical significance, especially after a multiple-comparison correction. To partially address this issue, isotropic "smoothing" or "filtering" of the image is often used. Another idea to increase the statistical power to detect widespread subtle abnormalities is to use an atlas-based analysis. In this method, a presegmented set of ROIs, which covers the entire brain, is overlaid on the normalized image to measure MR imaging parameters inside the ROIs. The automatically placed ROI is regarded as a filter to group voxels in anatomically reasonable way. Therefore, if one wants to achieve higher statistical power, one can increase the size of each ROI and reduce the total number of ROIs. In contrast, if one wants to know the precise localization of the abnormality, one can reduce the size of each ROI and increase the total number or ROIs. Again, the most extreme case is to use each voxel as an ROI. In either case, accurate image normalization is key for the quantitative image analysis.

NORMALIZATION-BASED NEONATAL BRAIN MR IMAGING ANALYSIS
Current Status of the Normalization-based MR Imaging Analysis

For MR imaging analysis of the adult or child's brain, normalization-based quantitative analysis methods are widely used, which is an effective way to characterize the anatomy of the normal population and pathologic changes.[30] However, for the neonate population, there are only a small number of studies using image normalization.[31–33] There are two reasons that hinder normalization-based MR imaging analysis of the neonatal brain. One is the lesser gray matter/white matter contrast in the neonatal brain. Transformation uses image contrasts to coregister the subjects' brain structures to that of the template. However, T1- and T2-weighted images from neonates have less contrast between each brain structure compared with the adult brain. The other is the lack of a standard neonatal atlas. For a study in a single institution, an arbitrarily selected image can be a template for the image normalization. However, if one wants to compare the results from multiple institutions, a "standardized" atlas on which to transform the image and report the area with significance with "common language" is needed. Because of the huge difference in image contrast between the neonatal and adult brain, one needs an atlas specifically made for the neonatal brain. For adult brain analysis, several brain atlases in standard space, such as Montreal Neurologic Institute space or Talairach space, are commonly used in the neuroimaging community. However, for neonatal studies, only a T1-weighted template created by averaging seven patients' brains (not normal control brains) and a T2-weighted template of 2 to 3 month olds (therefore, not a neonatal template) (http://www.unicog.org/main/pages.php?page=Infants) were available to the neuroimaging community until 2011.[32]

Core Components of the Normalization-based Analysis

The development of the neonatal brain is not uniform. Each brain structure develops at different times and rates. Especially for the white matter tracts, the myelination status and speed varies greatly. Therefore, each white matter structure must be identified accurately to avoid false-positive findings. For example, the superior longitudinal fasciculus is poorly myelinated in the neonatal brain, but the corticospinal tract is already myelinated to some extent. These two fibers are next to each other at the level of the centrum semi-ovale. If part of the superior longitudinal fasciculus is mislabeled as the corticospinal tract, one might conclude, wrongly, that the area is abnormal (less myelinated than usual). To avoid false-positive findings and to increase statistical power, the accuracy of the normalization, which guarantees each brain structure is correctly registered to the template space, is a crucial requirement.

Clear contrasts between each brain structure and appropriate normalization method are the two core components necessary for successful neonatal brain quantification. To satisfy these requirements, the authors created a neonatal brain atlas with multiple contrasts (JHU-neonate atlas, http://cmrm.med.jhmi.edu/cmrm/Data_neonate_atlas/atlas_neonate.htm), and combine the atlas with a state-of-the-art normalization method, large deformation diffeomorphic metric mapping (LDDMM).[34]

Multicontrast Atlas of the Neonatal Brain

There are various types of image contrasts that MR imaging can create, each with specific benefits. T2-weighted images have good contrast between brain tissue and the cerebrospinal fluid space, but lack contrasts inside the white matter area, which is treated as a large single compartment. DTI, however, has very rich contrasts within the white matter, enabling identification of various white matter structures, yet the brain boundary and ventricle shapes are obscure. In this way, T2 and DTI carry anatomic information that is spatially complementary. Conventionally, when one performs a brain transformation to an atlas, one needs

to choose one of the image contrasts to drive the registration algorithm. If one uses only one of the contrasts, the anatomic information is not sufficient to obtain satisfactory registration (**Fig. 5**). This is why there is a need to develop a multicontrast template for normalization, in which multiple contrasts are provided simultaneously.

The JHU-neonate atlas includes T1- and T2-weighted contrasts and DTI-derived contrasts. One hundred and twenty-two brain structures were parcellated in the atlas (**Fig. 6**) to create the "parcellation map," according to our previous publications.[35,36] The authors created both a population-averaged atlas and a single-subject atlas. The purpose of a population-averaged atlas is to determine the average shape and size of the neonatal brain. This atlas can be used as a template for brain normalization using linear transformations or nonlinear transformations with image "smoothing." However, as a result of averaging, the sharpness of the image contrast can be lost.[37] Therefore, a single-subject atlas, with the size adjusted to that of the population-averaged atlas, was also created, providing a template for highly elastic nonlinear transformations, which require sharp image features.[35]

CURRENT PRACTICAL ISSUES AND THE FUTURE OF NORMALIZATION-BASED NEONATAL BRAIN ANALYSIS

The authors are currently working on optimizing the MR imaging settings and the analysis tool (combination of the multicontrast neonatal brain atlas and LDDMM) to provide a good experimental environment for clinical researchers. Some of their experiences are described next.

Success Rate of the Neonatal Scan

Seventy normal-term neonates (within 48 hours of birth) were scanned using a Johns Hopkins University protocol on a 3-T magnet. Total time required for each neonate was approximately 30 minutes. Specifically, 5 minutes for each DTI acquisition with three repetitions to increase signal-to-noise ratio (15 minutes), two additional scans for TE = 42 milliseconds and 100 milliseconds to obtain a T2 map (6 minutes), and an MPRAGE image for anatomic reference (5 minutes) were obtained. To ensure that neonates were sleeping during the scan, neonates were well fed before the scan and were well wrapped with a blanket with the ears covered by earmuffs. The subjects were then placed in cushions that occupied spaces between the subject and the RF coil. Fifty-three of the 70 neonates slept through the scans without sedation (success rate of 75%).

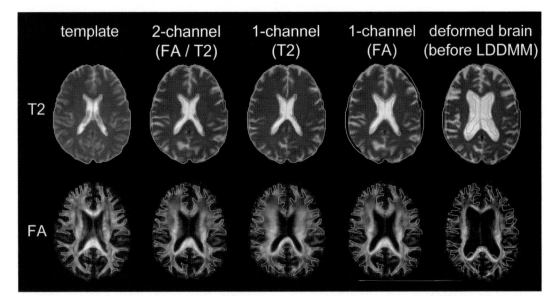

Fig. 5. The efficacy of dual-channel image registration. The blue line indicates the boundary of the brain (T2) and the white matter (FA) of the template. T2 and DTI carry contrasts in a spatially complementary manner. In this example, the atrophic brain with substantial ventricular enlargement is normalized to the template. When T2 is used to drive the transformation, the brain boundary and the ventricle of the patient become very similar to those of the template (T2), but the white matter structure is not similar to that of the template. If only the FA map is used, the white matter shape becomes very similar to the template, but the brain boundary is not matched (FA). By using both contrasts, the registration quality of the entire brain drastically improves (FA/T2). (*From* Ceritoglu C, Oishi K, Li X et al. Multi-contrast large deformation diffeomorphic metric mapping for diffusion tensor imaging. NeuroImage 2009;47:618; with permission.)

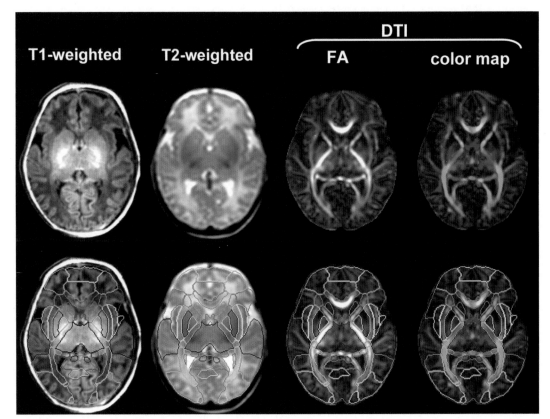

Fig. 6. The attempt to parcellate 122 brain structures from a full-term neonate. (*From* Oishi K, Mori S, Donohue PK, et al. Multi-contrast human neonatal brain atlas: application to normal neonate development analysis. NeuroImage 2011;56:8; with permission.)

Normalization Accuracy

As a preliminary analysis, the accuracy of normalization was compared using linear affine transformation, nonlinear transformation of SPM5, and of dual-channel LDDMM, which uses FA and T2 contrasts simultaneously (**Figs. 7** and **8**). To evaluate the registration quality, reliability analyses were performed to estimate kappa statistics, based on Landis and Koch.[38] According to the criteria, a kappa value of 0.11 to 0.2 is considered "slight," 0.21 to 0.4 is "fair," 0.41 to 0.60 is "moderate," 0.61 to 0.80 is "substantial," and 0.81 to 1 is "almost perfect" registration between a subject image and the atlas. Dual-channel LDDMM successfully improved the overall normalization accuracy to satisfy the requirement for neonatal brain MR imaging analysis in a structure-specific manner.

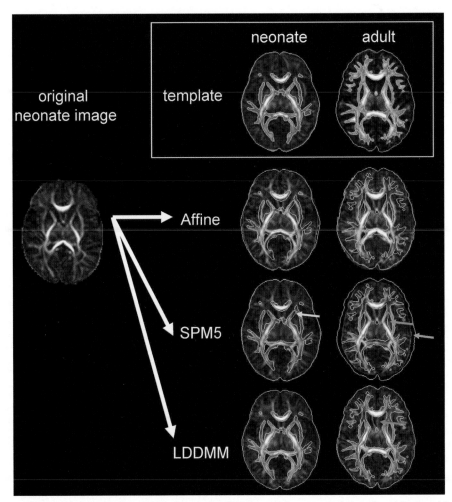

Fig. 7. The preliminary attempt to normalize a neonatal image to the neonatal template (single-subject image) and the adult template (Johns Hopkins University–Montreal Neurologic Institute template) using various normalizing methods. Normalized images (*two right columns*) were overlaid by the brain surface and WM areas of the templates, indicated by the blue contours. For all normalization methods, the neonatal template performed better than the adult template. The combination of the neonatal template and LDDMM achieved the best registration quality. Nonlinear transformation of SPM5 (http://www.fil.ion.ucl.ac.uk/spm) also demonstrated considerable registration quality with the neonatal template, although some misregistrations are indicated (eg, *yellow arrow*: the putamen was classified as the anterior limb of the internal capsule). This registration quality was better than that registered with the adult template (*pink arrow*: globus pallidum was classified as the internal capsule; *green arrow*: misregistration of the brain surface). LDDMM has enough transformation to normalize a neonatal image to the adult template, but the result was unreliable for the low FA structures, such as the septum (*red arrow*).

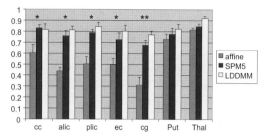

Fig. 8. Comparison of kappa values for each brain structure. LDDMM can improve registration accuracy in most structures, compared with linear (affine) transformation. One could also see the improvement in registration accuracy in the cingulum compared with the nonlinear transformation of SPM5. The data are from the average values of 10 full-term neonates. * Significant improvement compared with affine, P<.05 corrected after multiple comparisons. ** Significant improvement compared with both affine and SPM5, P<.05 corrected after multiple comparisons. The results indicate that this single-subject neonatal template is also applicable to the SPM, which is widely used in the neuroimaging community. alic, anterior limb of the internal capsule; cc, corpus callosum; cg, cingulum; ec, external capsule; plic, posterior limb of the internal capsule; Put, putamen; Thal, thalamus.

Future Application of the Normalization Based Neonatal MR Imaging Analysis

Future applications for this atlas include scientific investigations, such as determining the effects of prenatal events (hypoxia–ischemia, infections, or exposure to toxic substances) and the effects of preterm birth or low birth weight. This method enables one to perform whole-brain analysis, which is important for the visualization of structural specificity, but which was lacking in previous studies. These basic studies will lead to more clinical investigations, such as seeking imaging biomarkers for various neurologic disorders. The final goal is to use the measured value much like the results from blood tests, to make a diagnosis, evaluate the treatment, and predict future neurologic outcomes. Another goal is to create diagnostic criteria for the automated diagnosis of various diseases.

SUMMARY

This article describes the anatomic features of the neonatal brain and how one can quantify those features using structural MR imaging and DTI, which are complementary techniques. To maximize the potential of MR imaging for neonatal brain studies, the authors proposed to quantify both contrasts with a state-of-the-art diffeomorphic normalization method. Accurate and reproducible

MR imaging quantification achieved by this method is an initial step toward successful clinical research studies of the neonatal brain.

ACKNOWLEDGMENTS

The authors thank Dr Jon Skranes, Dr Tomas Ernst, and Dr Linda Chang for their helpful comments, and Mary McAllister for manuscript editing. This publication was made possible by grants from the National Institutes of Health (R21AG033774, P41RR015241, U24RR021382, P01EB00195, R01AG20012, and R01HD065955), and from the National Center for Research Resources grant G12-RR003061.

REFERENCES

1. Hack M, Fanaroff AA. Outcomes of children of extremely low birthweight and gestational age in the 1990's. Early Hum Dev 1999;53:193.
2. Hack M, Wilson-Costello D, Friedman H, et al. Neurodevelopment and predictors of outcomes of children with birth weights of less than 1000 g: 1992-1995. Arch Pediatr Adolesc Med 2000;154:725.
3. Perlman JM. Neurobehavioral deficits in premature graduates of intensive care: potential medical and neonatal environmental risk factors. Pediatrics 2001;108:1339.
4. Woodward LJ, Anderson PJ, Austin NC, et al. Neonatal MRI to predict neurodevelopmental outcomes in preterm infants. N Engl J Med 2006; 355:685.
5. Iida K, Takashima S, Ueda K. Immunohistochemical study of myelination and oligodendrocyte in infants with periventricular leukomalacia. Pediatr Neurol 1995;13:296.
6. Wiggins RC. Myelination: a critical stage in development. Neurotoxicology 1986;7:103.
7. Yakovlev PI, Lecours AR. Regional development of the brain in early life. Philadelphia: F.A. Davis; 1967.
8. Kinney HC, Brody BA, Kloman AS, et al. Sequence of central nervous system myelination in human infancy. II. Patterns of myelination in autopsied infants. J Neuropathol Exp Neurol 1988;47:217.
9. Barkovich AJ, Kjos BO, Jackson DE Jr, et al. Normal maturation of the neonatal and infant brain: MR imaging at 1.5 T. Radiology 1988;166:173.
10. Bird CR, Hedberg M, Drayer BP, et al. MR assessment of myelination in infants and children: usefulness of marker sites. AJNR Am J Neuroradiol 1989;10:731.
11. Christophe C, Muller MF, Baleriaux D, et al. Mapping of normal brain maturation in infants on phase-sensitive inversion–recovery MR images. Neuroradiology 1990;32:173.

12. Holland BA, Haas DK, Norman D, et al. MRI of normal brain maturation. AJNR Am J Neuroradiol 1986;7:201.

13. Baratti C, Barnett AS, Pierpaoli C. Comparative MR imaging study of brain maturation in kittens with T1, T2, and the trace of the diffusion tensor. Radiology 1999;210:133.

14. Miot-Noirault E, Barantin L, Akoka S, et al. T2 relaxation time as a marker of brain myelination: experimental MR study in two neonatal animal models. J Neurosci Methods 1997;72:5.

15. Neil JJ, Shiran SI, McKinstry RC, et al. Normal brain in human newborns: apparent diffusion coefficient and diffusion anisotropy measured by using diffusion tensor MR imaging. Radiology 1998;209:57.

16. Ono J, Kodaka R, Imai K, et al. Evaluation of myelination by means of the T2 value on magnetic resonance imaging. Brain Dev 1993;15:433.

17. Takeda K, Nomura Y, Sakuma H, et al. MR assessment of normal brain development in neonates and infants: comparative study of T1- and diffusion-weighted images. J Comput Assist Tomogr 1997;21:1.

18. Basser PJ, Mattiello J, LeBihan D. MR diffusion tensor spectroscopy and imaging. Biophys J 1994;66:259.

19. Hsu EW, Mori S. Analytical expressions for the NMR apparent diffusion coefficients in an anisotropic system and a simplified method for determining fiber orientation. Magn Reson Med 1995;34:194.

20. Mori S, Itoh R, Zhang J, et al. Diffusion tensor imaging of the developing mouse brain. Magn Reson Med 2001;46:18.

21. Pierpaoli C, Jezzard P, Basser PJ, et al. Diffusion tensor MR imaging of the human brain. Radiology 1996;201:637.

22. Pierpaoli C, Basser PJ. Toward a quantitative assessment of diffusion anisotropy. Magn Reson Med 1996;36:893.

23. Huppi PS, Maier SE, Peled S, et al. Microstructural development of human newborn cerebral white matter assessed in vivo by diffusion tensor magnetic resonance imaging. Pediatr Res 1998;44:584.

24. McKinstry RC, Mathur A, Miller JH, et al. Radial organization of developing preterm human cerebral cortex revealed by non-invasive water diffusion anisotropy MRI. Cereb Cortex 2002;12:1237.

25. Mukherjee P, Miller JH, Shimony JS, et al. Diffusion-tensor MR imaging of gray and white matter development during normal human brain maturation. AJNR Am J Neuroradiol 2002;23:1445.

26. De Vries LS, Groenendaal F, van Haastert IC, et al. Asymmetrical myelination of the posterior limb of the internal capsule in infants with periventricular haemorrhagic infarction: an early predictor of hemiplegia. Neuropediatrics 1999;30:314.

27. Roelants-van Rijn AM, Groenendaal F, Beek FJ, et al. Parenchymal brain injury in the preterm infant: comparison of cranial ultrasound, MRI and neurodevelopmental outcome. Neuropediatrics 2001;32:80.

28. Hayakawa K, Kanda T, Hashimoto K, et al. MR imaging of spastic diplegia. The importance of corpus callosum. Acta Radiol 1996;37:830.

29. Inder TE, Warfield SK, Wang H, et al. Abnormal cerebral structure is present at term in premature infants. Pediatrics 2005;115:286.

30. Oishi K, Konishi J, Mori S, et al. Reduced fractional anisotropy in early-stage cerebellar variant of multiple system atrophy. J Neuroimaging 2009;19:127.

31. Kazemi K, Ghadimi S, Abrishami-Moghaddam H, et al. Neonatal probabilistic models for brain, CSF and skull using T1-MRI data: preliminary results. Conf Proc IEEE Eng Med Biol Soc 2008;2008:3892.

32. Kazemi K, Moghaddam HA, Grebe R, et al. A neonatal atlas template for spatial normalization of whole-brain magnetic resonance images of newborns: preliminary results. Neuroimage 2007;37:463.

33. Shi F, Fan Y, Tang S, et al. Neonatal brain image segmentation in longitudinal MRI studies. Neuroimage 2010;49:391.

34. Oishi K, Mori S, Donohue P, et al. Multi-contrast human neonatal brain atlas: application to normal neonate development analysis. NeuroImage 2011;56:8.

35. Oishi K, Faria A, Jiang H, et al. Atlas-based whole brain white matter analysis using large deformation diffeomorphic metric mapping: application to normal elderly and Alzheimer's disease participants. Neuroimage 2009;46:486.

36. Oishi K, Zilles K, Amunts K, et al. Human brain white matter atlas: identification and assignment of common anatomical structures in superficial white matter. Neuroimage 2008;43:447.

37. Mori S, Oishi K, Jiang H, et al. Stereotaxic white matter atlas based on diffusion tensor imaging in an ICBM template. Neuroimage 2008;40:570.

38. Landis JR, Koch GG. An application of hierarchical kappa-type statistics in the assessment of majority agreement among multiple observers. Biometrics 1977;33:363.

Head Ultrasound and MR Imaging in the Evaluation of Neonatal Encephalopathy: Competitive or Complementary Imaging Studies?

Monica Epelman, MD[a],*, Alan Daneman, MD, FRCPC[b],
Nancy Chauvin, MD[a], Wolfgang Hirsch, MD[c]

KEYWORDS

- Encephalopathy • Hypoxic–ischemic injury • Neonate
- Sonography • Ultrasound • MR imaging

Neonatal encephalopathy (NE) is a major cause of mortality and morbidity in newborns. NE occurs in 1 to 6 per 1000 live full-term births and is the most important cause of brain damage in the newborn. The consequences are potentially devastating, because it can lead to mortality or severe disability.[1]

This article discusses and illustrates the ultrasound (US) findings present in infants with NE and correlates them with the findings present on MR imaging when appropriate. Although MR imaging has become more widely used and has gained widespread acceptance in the evaluation of NE in recent years, US continues to be the primary screening imaging modality used for the evaluation of the neonatal brain. In many neonates, the diagnosis of brain abnormalities has been made using cranial US. It is a noninvasive, inexpensive, and portable imaging modality that allows examinations to be performed without requiring transport of the infant. The anterior fontanelle provides a convenient sonographic window that allows excellent imaging of many regions of the brain.

Throughout the article, the clinical use of linear US images that are obtained with high-frequency linear array transducers is emphasized. Also discussed is how Doppler imaging and additional windows can be used to improve diagnostic accuracy. Linear US images are a useful adjunct to conventional US and enable further characterization of the architecture of the brain parenchyma, pathologic conditions, and in some instances more precise anatomic localization and diagnoses.

---

[a] Department of Radiology, The Children's Hospital of Philadelphia, 34th Street and Civic Center Boulevard, Philadelphia, PA 19104, USA
[b] Department of Diagnostic Imaging, The Hospital for Sick Children, University of Toronto, Toronto, ON, Canada
[c] Universität Leipzig, Selbstständige Abteilung für Pädiatrische Radiologie, Liebigstrasse 20A, 04103 Leipzig, Germany
* Corresponding author.
E-mail address: monica_epelman@hotmail.com

Magn Reson Imaging Clin N Am 20 (2012) 93–115
doi:10.1016/j.mric.2011.08.012

CLINICAL FEATURES OF NE

NE is clinically defined as a "syndrome of disturbed neurologic function in the earliest days after birth in the term infant, manifested by difficulty with initiating and maintaining respiration, depression of tone and reflexes, subnormal level of consciousness and often seizures"[2]; whereas hypoxic–ischemic injury (HII) is defined as NE with intrapartum hypoxia in the absence of any other abnormality. HII is characterized by a distinctive encephalopathy that evolves from lethargy to hyperexcitability to stupor during the first 3 days of life. Neonates with HII are usually born at term, but the condition also occurs in premature neonates. HII may be difficult to diagnose in premature infants, especially those with very low birth weight, because the obvious signs are absent or because the symptoms that are present are attributed to developmental immaturity.[1,3,4] Involvement of multiple additional organs is a characteristic feature of HII. HII may present with multiorgan dysfunction and severely depressed cardiovascular function, particularly if it is severe.[5,6] Patients may have severe pulmonary hypertension requiring assisted ventilation. Renal (eg, anuria or oliguria), hepatic (eg, abnormal liver function tests), and gastrointestinal injury (eg, delayed gastric emptying and poor peristalsis)

are also common, although they do not occur immediately.[7,8] Notably, the presence of renal dysfunction in association with an abnormal neurologic clinical examination in infants with HII is associated with a poor long-term neurodevelopmental outcome.[6]

According to the guidelines of the American College of Obstetricians and Gynecologists (ACOG) and the American Academy of Pediatrics (AAP),[9] the following four criteria must be present for a diagnosis of HII to be made: (1) evidence of metabolic acidosis (pH <7.0 and a base deficit of ≥12 mmol/L); (2) early onset of severe or moderate NE in infants born at greater than or equal to 34 weeks' gestation; (3) quadriplegic or dyskinetic cerebral palsy (CP); and (4) exclusion of other identifiable etiologies, such as trauma, infection, a coagulation disorder, or a genetic disorder. However, although CP is frequently attributed to asphyxia, most cases of CP are not associated with severe perinatal asphyxia, and vice versa not all cases of perinatal asphyxia result in CP.[6,10,11] It is also believed that some infants who develop HII may have experienced asphyxia or brain hypoxia remote from the time of delivery but exhibit the signs and symptoms of hypoxic encephalopathy at the time of birth.[9,12]

More than 10 years ago, a case-control study performed in Western Australia[13,14] concluded

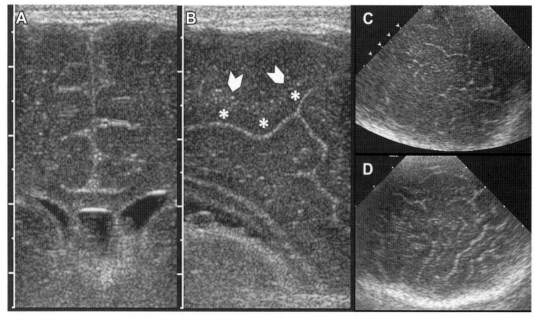

Fig. 1. (A) Magnified coronal US image, (B) magnified sagittal US image, and (C, D) peripheral angled views show normal echogenicity of the gray–white matter differentiation. The sulci appear as curvilinear echogenic lines. The central portions of the gyri constitute the most echogenic portions of the white matter (arrowheads) and the echogenicity decreases gradually as one moves toward the gray matter (asterisks). The boundary between the gray and white matter is ill-defined under normal conditions.

that there was no evidence of intrapartum asphyxia in more than 70% of cases of NE. They found that the causes of NE are heterogeneous and many occur before birth. The antepartum risk factors for NE include (1) low socioeconomic status; (2) advanced maternal age; (3) a family history of seizures; (4) maternal thyroid disease; (5) maternal hypertension; (6) vaginal bleeding; (7) conception after infertility treatment; (8) in utero viral illness; (9) abnormal placenta; (10) postterm delivery; and (11) intrauterine growth restriction, with the latter being the strongest risk factor. Only a small fraction of NE is caused by HII, and it has been associated with intrapartum risk factors, such as forceps delivery, breech extraction, cord prolapse, abruptio placentae, and maternal fever.[13,14]

In 2003, Cowan and colleagues[15] found that more than 90% of 360 term infants without known genetic syndromes or major congenital defects who underwent MR imaging within the first 2 weeks of life and who developed NE, seizures, or both had MR imaging evidence of brain injury at or near the time of delivery. However, these authors could not distinguish between brain injuries acquired during versus just before delivery.

More recently, several investigators[3,16] have emphasized the importance of maternal infection during pregnancy as a major risk factor for CP in term and preterm infants. In a review by Graham and colleagues[17] published in 2008, the authors concluded that despite the existence of objective criteria for grading of NE, investigators often use different definitions of intrapartum HII, which results in variations in different institutions' rates of NE. Nonetheless, regardless of the definition applied, the incidence of HII in developed countries was 2.5 per 1000 live births, and only 14.5%

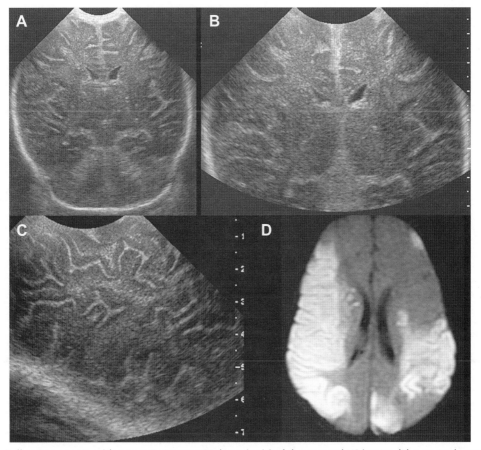

Fig. 2. Full-term neonate with group B streptococcal meningitis. (*A*) A coronal US image, (*B*) a coronal magnified view, and (*C*) a sagittal peripheral angled view showing abnormal GWMD. The sulci are thick and hyperechogenic. The white matter appears hyperechogenic relative to the hypoechoic gray matter. The GWMD is accentuated. These findings are consistent with mild to moderate brain edema and triggered further MR imaging investigation in this encephalopathic neonate. (*D*) Axial MR diffusion-weighted image shows bilateral middle cerebral artery territory infarcts. In this case, the MR imaging revealed more extensive and more florid injury than was present on US.

of CP cases in the reviewed studies were associated with intrapartum hypoxia–ischemia. Therefore, the term NE is favored over HII unless all of the ACOG and AAP[9] criteria are known to be met. It also should be noted that the cause of CP remains incompletely understood.[18,19]

Patients' clinical manifestations and course vary depending on the severity of their NE. Although several scoring systems exist,[20,21] the staging system created by Sarnat and Sarnat[2] is the most widely used. It recognizes three stages of NE and correlates them with clinical outcomes. At one end of the spectrum, Sarnat stage 1, or mild encephalopathy, is characterized by irritability, poor feeding, hyperreflexia, and an exaggerated

Moro reflex and has no long term-sequelae. On the other end of the spectrum, patients with Sarnat stage 3, or severe encephalopathy, have seizures and usually require ventilatory support. These patients usually have poor outcomes.

NEUROPATHOLOGIC FEATURES OF PERINATAL BRAIN INJURIES

There are four major patterns of hypoxic–ischemic brain lesions: (1) parasagittal brain injury, (2) periventricular leukomalacia (PVL), (3) selective neuronal necrosis (SNN), and (4) focal or multifocal ischemic brain lesions.[6,22,23]

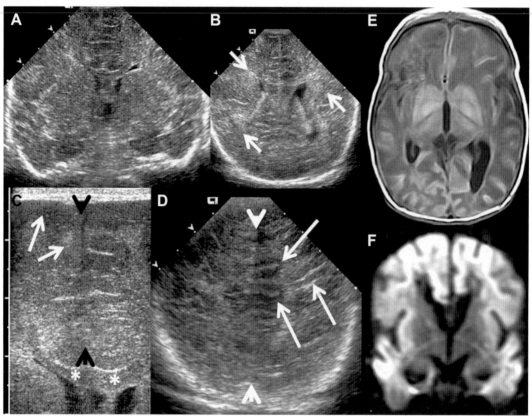

Fig. 3. A 6-day-old, ex-35-week premature neonate with seizures and HII. (A, B) Coronal US images showing patchy areas (arrows) of increased echogenicity, right greater than left. (C) Magnified coronal US image obtained with a linear transducer depicts these abnormalities more clearly. There is complete loss of GWMD on the right and partial loss of GWMD on the left within the areas adjacent to the interhemispheric fissure. The asterisks denote the corpus callosum. The interhemispheric fissure is indistinct (arrowheads). The cortex on the right appears swollen, echogenic, and thickened (arrows). (D) A coronal US image obtained through the convexity reveals a mixed pattern of loss and accentuation of the GWMD. GWMD is lost in the right hemisphere, whereas it is accentuated in some areas of the left hemisphere (arrows). The interhemispheric fissure is blurred (arrowheads). Collectively, these findings are more severe than those in Fig. 2 and indicate moderate to severe brain edema or ischemia. (E) This axial T1-weighted image shows findings of laminar necrosis and a diffuse abnormal signal in the basal ganglia. (F) This coronal diffusion-weighted image shows extensive areas of restricted diffusion. Although the US images show some abnormalities, the changes on MR imaging are more extensive and more florid.

Parasagittal Brain Injury

This condition usually occurs in term neonates. It is classically bilateral, symmetric, and affects the parasagittal portions of the cerebral convexities corresponding to the "watershed" areas between the territories of the anterior, middle, and posterior cerebral arteries.[22,23] This type of damage is associated with chronic, possibly repetitive ischemic insults[24]; mild to moderate hypotension[25]; and reflects the so-called "prolonged partial asphyxia."[26] In these cases, brain injury occurs secondary to insufficient perfusion to the watershed areas between the main cerebral arteries during periods of ischemia. This type of injury mainly affects the motor cortex (especially the portion responsible for proximal extremity function) and its clinical manifestations tend to include seizures, hypotension, or both. The upper extremities are often more severely affected than the lower extremities. These patients present with spastic quadriplegia and seizure disorders later in life. Their cognitive outcome is unpredictable.[6,22,26]

Periventricular Leukomalacia

PVL is the most common injury in preterm neonates and is caused by the anatomic characteristics of the brain's circulation related to gestational age. Before 32 weeks of gestation, blood vessels penetrate the cortex from the pial surface. Fetuses of this age have short penetrators (which end in the subcortical white matter) and long penetrators (which extend deeper into the brain). This results in relatively poor vascularization of the periventricular white matter, which predisposes premature infants to ischemic injury.[27] The areas that are the most prone to damage include the

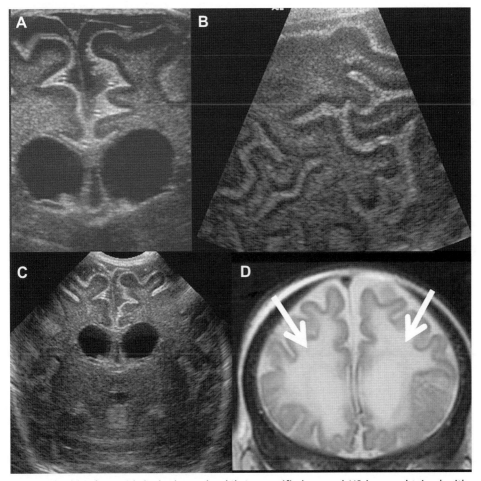

Fig. 4. A 6-month-old infant with leukodystrophy. (*A*) A magnified coronal US image obtained with a linear transducer, (*B*) a magnified sagittal peripheral angled view, and (*C*) a coronal US image reveal accentuation of the GWMD. (*D*) Coronal T2-weighted MR image shows abnormal signal in the frontal white matter (*arrows*). Abnormal GWMD is a sensitive, but not a specific, finding of NE.

periventricular white matter that is dorsal and lateral to the external angles of the lateral ventricles, particularly the centrum semiovale and the optic (trigone and occipital horns) and acoustic (temporal horn) radiations. Because the lower-extremity axons of the corticospinal tract, which are periventricular in location, course medially to upper-extremity axons, these patients present later in life with spastic diplegia (ie, impaired motor function that affects the lower extremities most severely). Visual field disorders are also characteristic of PVL because of damage that occurs within the optic radiations. With more severe brain injury,

spastic quadriplegia with associated visual and cognitive deficits may also be observed.[6,22,27]

Selective Neuronal Necrosis

SNN is the most common pattern associated with hypoxic–ischemic events and usually coexists with all of the other patterns. The site of the injury depends on the severity of the insult and gestational age of the neonate. The long-term sequelae of this type of injury include mental retardation, spastic quadriparesis, and seizures. Choreoathetosis and dystonia may be seen if the thalamus

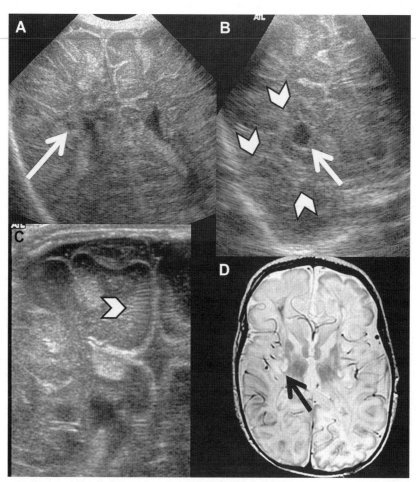

Fig. 5. A 10-day-old male infant with molybdenum cofactor deficiency and seizures. (*A*) This axial US image reveals a heterogeneous appearance of the brain parenchyma and raised suspicion of a small parenchymal cyst (*arrow*). (*B*) Magnified axial focused US image of the periphery of the brain reveals a mixed pattern of accentuation and loss of the gray–white matter boundary. The cyst (*arrow*) is better delineated on this dedicated image and is situated in close proximity to the Sylvian fissure (*arrowheads*). (*C*) Magnified coronal US image shows an abnormal striated appearance of the cortex adjacent to the interhemispheric fissure (*arrowhead*). (*D*) Axial T2-weighted image reveals extensive areas of severe brain edema bilaterally with loss of GWMD. A cyst is noted on the right (*arrow*). Extensive areas of restricted diffusion were appreciated on DWI (image not shown). Although the MR imaging changes demonstrated are more extensive and florid, US was an important initial modality, which depicted enough brain parenchymal abnormalities to prompt the MR imaging study.

and basal ganglia are involved. Of note, the basal ganglia seem to be particularly sensitive to hypoxia. Bulbar and pseudobulbar palsy can occur if the brainstem and tegmentum are affected. Hypoperfusion with subsequent reperfusion injury and glutamate-induced injury are involved in the pathogenesis of SNN.[6,22,23] The four major patterns of injury include (1) diffuse, (2) cerebral cortex–deep gray matter, (3) deep gray matter–brainstem, and (4) pontosubicular injury.

Diffuse neuronal injury

This type of SNN occurs after severe, very prolonged hypoxic–ischemic insults in both term and premature infants and affects nearly all neurons in the neuroaxis. It most frequently affects the cortex, hippocampus, cerebellum, and anterior horn cells of the spinal cord. Within the cortex, the injury is more prominent in the watershed zones and more marked in the depth of the sulci than in the gyri.[22,23] With more severe injuries, the more differentiated visual (calcarine) cortex and the perirolandic cortex may be damaged.

Cerebral cortex–deep gray matter

This type of SNN occurs mainly in term neonates after moderate to severe, usually prolonged hypoxic–ischemic insults. Injury is generally bilateral and typically affects the dorsolateral putamen and ventrolateral thalami. This combination is typical of HII in the term neonate.

Deep gray matter–brainstem

This type of SNN occurs mainly in term neonates after severe, prolonged insults that are fairly abrupt in onset. Although injury to the basal ganglia and thalamus occurs in roughly 75% of these patients, only 15% to 20% of neonates with HII exhibit involvement of the deep gray matter and brainstem as the prevailing lesion that is present, and only a portion of these evolve to

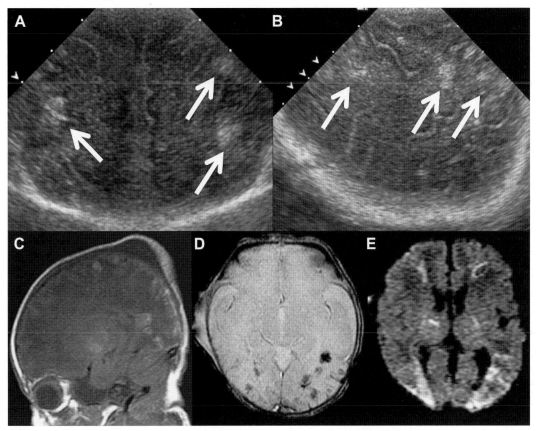

Fig. 6. A 2 week old with *Serratia* septicemia. (*A*) Coronal and (*B*) sagittal US images focused on the periphery reveal multiple, focal ill-defined, patchy areas of increased echogenicity (*arrows*) within the subcortical white matter. (*C*) Sagittal T1-weighted image shows multiple patchy foci of hemorrhage and evidence of cortical laminar necrosis in the parieto-occipital areas. (*D*) Axial gradient-echo image shows multiple foci of susceptibility consistent with blood products. (*E*) Axial DWI shows restricted diffusion in some of these areas, indicating that there is a component of ischemia present.

"status marmoratus." Status marmoratus is so-named because of the marbled appearance acquired by the affected structures (particularly the putamen) after this type of injury. It is characterized by neuronal loss, gliosis, and hypermyelination. The complete pathologic picture is not apparent until at least 8 months after birth, although the insult occurs in the perinatal period. The clinical condition manifests later in life with cognitive deficits and movement disorders, including choreoathetosis and dystonia, which may not be apparent until 1 to 4 years of age.[22,24]

Pontosubicular injury

This type of SNN affects the neurons of the basis pontis and the subiculum of the hippocampus. This type of injury occurs mainly in preterm neonates and is strongly associated with PVL. Clinically, it is associated with hypoxia–ischemia, hypocarbia, and hyperoxia.[22,28]

Focal or Multifocal Ischemic Brain Lesions

This form of injury is unusual before the 28th week of gestation. Its incidence increases with gestational age and most commonly occurs as a result of postnatal events. It mainly affects the middle cerebral artery territory, and it affects the left middle cerebral artery more often than it affects the right. When venous structures are affected, superior sagittal sinus thrombosis is the most common causative lesion. The major causes of these lesions include perinatal asphyxia, infection, trauma, and coagulation disorders. However, the etiology of this type of injury remains unknown in roughly half of patients.[22]

Differentiation between these various types of brain lesions, especially between focal or multifocal necrosis, parasagittal injury, and PVL, can be challenging, and in many cases these patterns of injury coexist.[22,23]

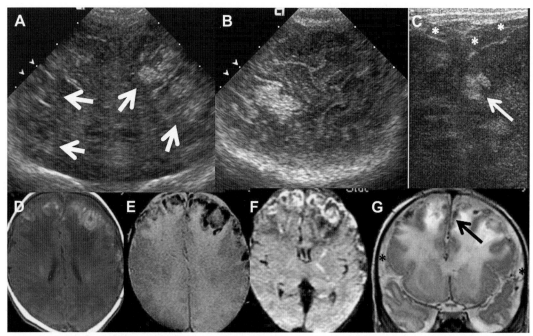

Fig. 7. A 20-day-old full-term neonate with sepsis, meningitis, and seizures. (*A*) These coronal and (*B*) sagittal focused US images reveal multiple, extensive foci of increased echogenicity in the bilateral frontal lobes (*arrows*), left greater than right. (*C*) Magnified coronal US image reveals a swollen cortex with areas in which the GWMD is accentuated and others in which it is lost. In addition, a few hemorrhagic cortical foci are seen (*arrow*). The fluid in the extraaxial spaces appears turbid (*asterisks*). (*D*) Corresponding axial T1-weighted image shows extensive areas of T1-shortening. (*E*) Axial gradient-echo image demonstrates multiple foci of susceptibility in the bilateral frontal lobes, left greater than right, which is consistent with hemorrhagic products and corresponding to the US images. (*F*) Axial DWI reveals restricted diffusion in some of these areas. Note the restricted diffusion that is present in the left internal capsule. (*G*) Coronal T2-weighted image demonstrates extensive frontal lobe edema bilaterally and foci of hemorrhage, one of which (*arrow*) corresponds to the focus noted on (*C*). Overall, these findings are consistent with extensive hemorrhagic necrosis and cavitary changes involving the frontal lobes, bilaterally. This is thought to be secondary to the underlying infectious etiology. Note the small bilateral subdural effusions (*asterisks*) and mild midline shift that are present.

At the molecular level, it has recently been postulated that HII occurs in two steps in the mature fetal brain: ischemia and reperfusion. The first is believed to be the result of an acute reduction in umbilical or uterine circulation. Recently, it has been postulated that a considerable proportion of neuronal injury occurs during the second phase of neuronal cell damage, the reperfusion phase. This is believed to result from several different types of inflammatory reactions in conjunction with the inhibition of protein synthesis, which eventually leads to the induction of neuronal apoptosis (programmed cell death).[23,29] There are also increasing data showing an association between HII and ascending intrauterine infections either before or after birth, possibly caused by endotoxin-mediated cytokine release. Furthermore, it is believed to be a synergistic effect between infection and HII.[3,23,30]

US CHARACTERISTICS OF NE

The classic imaging findings of acute HII have been widely described and typically include focally

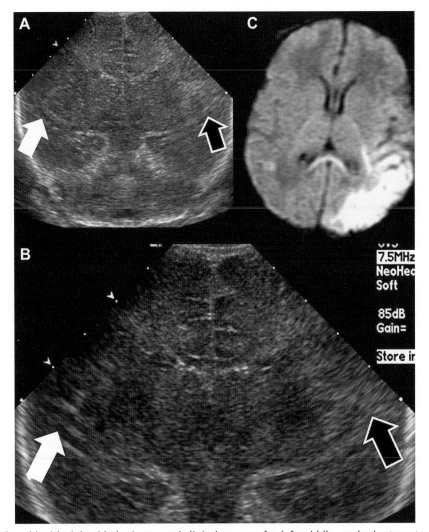

Fig. 8. A 6 day old with right-sided seizures and clinical concern for left middle cerebral artery stroke. (*A*) This coronal US image shows a faint, ill-defined area of abnormally increased echogenicity in the parenchyma adjacent to the left Sylvian fissure. Also note the indistinctness of the Sylvian fissure on the left side (*black arrow*) compared with the contralateral side (*white arrow*), a finding that should raise suspicion of an underlying abnormality. (*B*) A focused view of the area reveals similar findings to (*A*). There is a more patchy area of faintly increased echogenicity within the subcortical white matter adjacent to the left Sylvian fissure. (*C*) This axial DWI reveals restricted diffusion within the left temporal–parietal area in the distribution of the distal left middle cerebral artery consistent with ischemic injury.

or diffusely increased echogenicity of the brain parenchyma and a slit-like appearance of the ventricles with obliteration of the extracerebral cerebral spinal fluid spaces and the interhemispheric fissure.[31–33] However, in the authors' experience, these findings are usually seen only in advanced cases of NE. In less severe cases, the findings are less conspicuous and can only be appreciated when linear or magnified US images are obtained.[34] This is not a novel or exotic finding, because as far back as 1994, Eken and colleagues[35] reported on the improved use of high-resolution US images obtained with high MHz transducers compared with conventional US images. They compared US findings obtained with high MHz probes with autopsy findings in 20

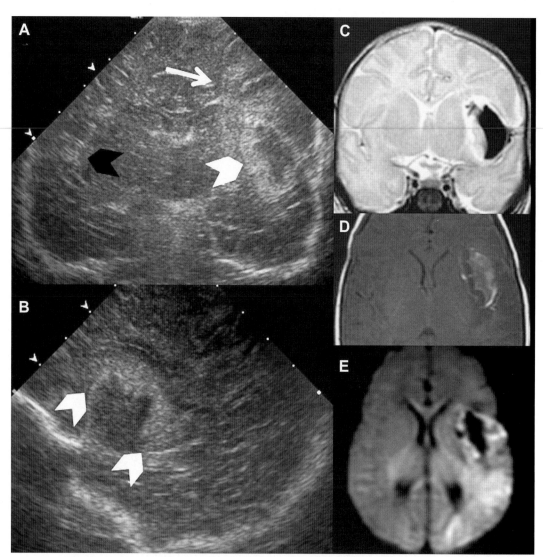

Fig. 9. A 1 day old with a history of meconium aspiration, HII, and seizures. (A) These coronal and (B) sagittal US images reveal an area of ill-defined increased echogenicity adjacent to the left Sylvian fissure (*white arrowheads*). The left Sylvian fissure is indistinct compared with the Sylvian fissure on the contralateral side (*black arrowhead*). The white matter adjacent to this area shows increased echogenicity consistent with edema (*arrow in A*) and there is accentuation of the GWMD compared with the contralateral side. (C) Coronal T2-weighted image, (D) axial T1-weighted image, and (E) axial DWI show an area of abnormal signal in the left Sylvian region that is dark in the T2-weighted images and mildly bright on the T1-weighted images, consistent with an acute hematoma in the left Sylvian fissure area. There are areas of restricted diffusion in both hemispheres, left greater than right, that are consistent with ischemia and infarction. The aforementioned left Sylvian fissure bleed is probably a hemorrhagic transformation of an area of ischemia and infarction. The MR image showed the findings more extensively and floridly than the US.

patients using a high-resolution 10-MHz transducer to better depict pathology in several locations in the brain. They found that this technique was particularly useful for identifying lesions in the thalamus, and that it was able to do so with a sensitivity of 100% and a specificity of 83%. This technique was also excellent at depicting lesions in other regions of the brain. The authors found a sensitivity and specificity of 100% and 83% for cortical lesions and 77% and 100% for white matter lesions, respectively.

This article is based on a review of the existing medical literature and the authors' 29-month experience with 76 neonatal patients in whom brain US and MR imaging were prospectively obtained within 2 hours of one another.[36] This cohort of patients forms the basis for the current discussion, with an emphasis placed on subtle, lesser known findings that may improve the diagnosis and characterization of NE. The main purposes of this article are to increase readers' awareness of the subtle findings on linear or magnified US images (which are usually more conspicuous on MR imaging and may be associated with the presence of severe disease) that may allow a diagnosis of NE to be made; and to emphasize the technical factors that may optimize US imaging of these patients. It is well beyond the scope of this article,

however, to review the detailed management of NE or to describe in detail the MR imaging findings that can be observed in patients with this condition.

In the authors' experience, the head US findings associated with NE may be divided into three main groups to allow for better characterization of the lesions that are present:

1. Peripheral brain
   a. Gray–white matter differentiation
   b. Cortical abnormalities
   c. Subcortical white matter
2. Central findings
   a. Basal ganglia
   b. Brainstem and posterior fossa
   c. Periventricular white matter
   d. Ventricular size
3. Doppler findings
   a. Resistive indices
   b. Hyperemia
   c. Sinus vein patency

PERIPHERAL US FINDINGS
Gray–white Matter Differentiation

Differentiation between gray and white matter is possible with the use of high-frequency linear

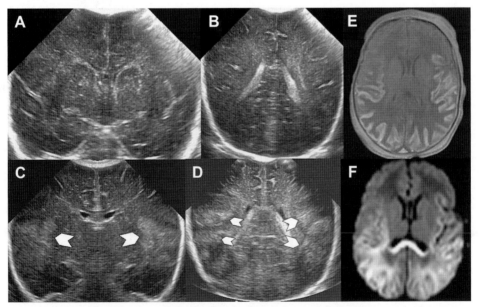

Fig. 10. A 2 week old with herpes simplex virus encephalitis, coagulopathy, and seizures. (*A, B*) These coronal US images show mild accentuation of the GWMD consistent with mild brain edema. The ventricles appear small. (*C, D*) Images obtained 2 days later because of the patient's clinical deterioration reveal the interval development patchy areas of abnormally increased cortical echogenicity bilaterally. The previously distinct Sylvian fissures are now indistinct and appear swollen (*arrowheads* in *C*). The previously noted sulci at the level of the bilateral atria are now indistinct and manifest heterogeneous echogenicity (*arrowheads* in *D*). (*E*) Axial T1-weighted image shows extensive areas of cortical laminar necrosis. (*F*) Axial DWI shows extensive areas of cortical and subcortical ischemic injury.

array transducers.[34,37,38] The sulci demonstrate moderately high echogenicity as opposed to the gyri. Both gray and white matter are relatively hypoechoic and homogeneous in appearance, and the cortical gray matter is only slightly more hypoechoic than the adjacent subcortical white matter. Thus, the boundary between gray and white matter is subtle within the normal brain (**Fig. 1**).

Accentuation of gray–white matter differentiation (GWMD) is an early sign of brain edema (**Fig. 2**).[34,37,38] As edema worsens, the classically described appearance of slit-like ventricles, sulcal effacement, and either generalized or patchy increases in the echogenicity of the brain parenchyma is seen.[32,33] In advanced cases GWMD is lost (**Fig. 3**).

The differential diagnosis for this pattern of accentuation of GWMD includes congenital infections and leukodystrophies, such as Canavan disease and Alexander disease (**Fig. 4**).[39,40]

The authors found that all of their patients with NE[36] had evidence of increased GWMD on US, making it the most sensitive indicator of NE, although it was a relatively nonspecific finding. The more severe the accentuation of the GWMD on US the more severe the findings encountered on diffusion-weighted imaging (DWI). GWMD can be easily assessed either with linear array transducers in the coronal plane or with focused, magnified views of the periphery of the brain in the coronal and parasagittal planes. These focused views are particularly useful for evaluating this parameter.

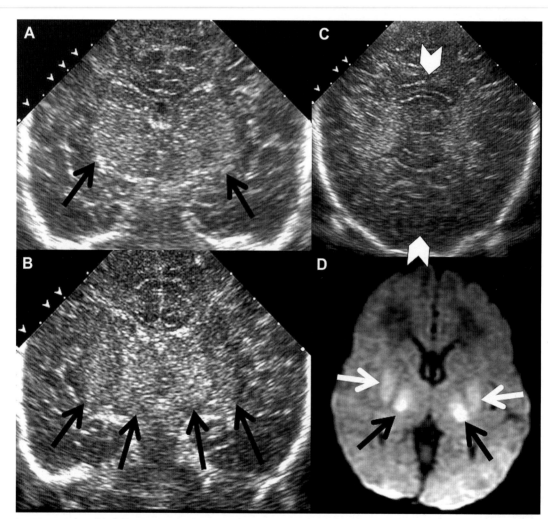

Fig. 11. A 2-day-old, fullterm neonate with a history of a profound hypoxic–ischemic injury. (*A, B*) Coronal US images show slit-like ventricles and mild, diffuse increased echogenicity of the basal ganglia (*arrows*). (*C*) Focused, peripheral view of the convexity shows accentuation of the GWMD and blurring of the interhemispheric fissure (*arrowheads*). (*D*) Axial DWI shows restricted diffusion in the bilateral posterior putamen (*white arrows*) and ventrolateral thalami (*black arrows*).

Caution should be taken in patients who have increased amounts of subarachnoid fluid (eg, patients with atrophy or benign macrocephaly of infancy), because the multiple interfaces that are present between the fluid and sulci may artificially thicken the sulci resulting in a pseudoaccentuation of GWMD.

Cortical Abnormalities

Cortical laminar necrosis has been associated with cortical high signal on T1-weighted images.[24] This abnormality is most commonly seen near the central sulcus, interhemispheric fissure, and insula.[24] It is important to note that US evidence of cortical injury has not been previously described in patients with NE. The authors found cortical abnormalities in 17 of their patients,[36] evidenced by abnormally increased or decreased GWMD with additional mild focal thickening and increased echogenicity of the gray matter. The gray matter also showed focal areas of heterogeneous echogenicity or displayed subtle linear transverse echogenicities of uncertain significance, which probably occurred because of cerebral edema and brain swelling (**Figs. 5** and **6**). In some of these patients cortical laminar necrosis was noted on MR imaging.

Subcortical White Matter

Although it is generally believed that the periphery of the brain cannot be adequately assessed by US,

with the use of transducers with high near-field resolution and the addition of angled views this limitation can be easily overcome.[37] These advances may help not only with the assessment of the GWMD, but also with the evaluation of the subcortical white matter, which may exhibit areas of focal abnormalities that can be easily overlooked if these techniques are not used (**Figs. 5–10**).

CENTRAL US FINDINGS
Basal Ganglia

Abnormalities of the basal ganglia and thalami are commonly observed after profound asphyxia. This is believed to be related to the increased metabolic rate in these areas, which are actively undergoing myelination at the time of delivery in term neonates.[24] The normal echogenicity of the basal ganglia and thalami in neonates is intermediate to low. Although it is believed that US underestimates the extent of injury to the deep gray matter,[33] thalamic injury may be recognized as a subtle or pronounced increase in echogenicity that may be unilateral or bilateral and is usually diffuse (**Figs. 11** and **12**).[4,41,42] This is particularly true when linear US images or magnified views that are dedicated to these areas are used. This increase in echogenicity is believed to be either secondary to redistribution of the cerebral blood flow from the anterior to the posterior circulation or caused by a diffuse decrease in echogenicity of the rest of

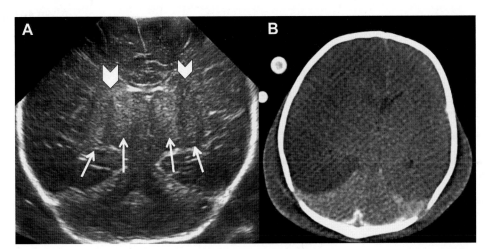

Fig. 12. A 1-month-old infant on extracorporeal membrane oxygenation with worsening clinical status. (*A*) Coronal US image shows slit-like ventricles, diffusely increased echogenicity of the basal ganglia (*arrows*), and a 5-mm midline shift right to left. Note the relatively hypoechoic appearance of the bilateral internal capsules (*arrowheads*). (*B*) Unenhanced CT scan reveals diffuse, severe cerebral edema, right greater than left. Note the relative increase in density of the cerebellum compared with the brain hemispheres. This is consistent with the so-called "reversal sign." Extracorporeal membrane oxygenation cannulas are present in the upper left corner of the image. Overall, the findings are consistent with a global hypoxic–ischemic insult.

the brain parenchyma secondary to edema, decreased blood flow, or encephalomalacia.[32]

Leijser and colleagues[43] noted that the visualization of the internal capsule as a hypoechoic linear area adjacent to the hyperechoic basal ganglia and white matter was highly predictive of abnormal motor function later in life (see **Fig. 12A**).

One should be cautious when assessing the thalami via the posterior fossa approach because Schlesinger and colleagues[44] found that foci of increased echogenicity can also be noted in patients without NE. This finding could be the result of anisotropism related to the interaction between the US beam and the different intrathalamic structures or caused by partial volume averaging between the posterior limb of the internal capsule and lateral portions of the thalamus. The authors found it useful to obtain magnified images via the anterior fontanelle to confirm or exclude these abnormalities in patients with these US findings.

Brainstem and Posterior Fossa

The cerebral peduncles and the quadrigeminal plates are paired hypoechoic, lenticular, wing-like structures that can be easily evaluated by way of the transmastoid retroauricular approach. This approach has been found to be far superior to the anterior fontanelle approach.[45–47] Brainstem lesions, although commonly seen in the setting of profound HII, are believed to be elusive on US studies. However, by obtaining dedicated views through the transmastoid retroauricular approach, focal areas of abnormal echogenicity that are suggestive of ischemic injury may be observed (**Fig. 13**). Neonatal brainstem tumors, particularly pontine gliomas, may present with NE.[48] On US pontine gliomas may appear as an enlarged echogenic pons resulting in hydrocephalus (**Fig. 14**). Of note, a proportion of these tumors are believed to resolve spontaneously.[48] Cerebellar injury primarily affects very preterm infants. Transmastoid views are a useful adjunct in this setting

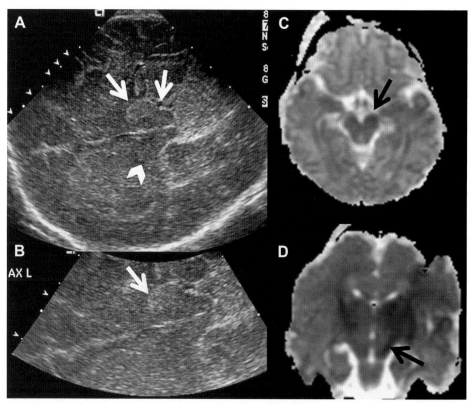

Fig. 13. A full-term neonate with HII and a right-sided focus of activity on EEG. (*A*) This axial image obtained through the midbrain via a left transmastoid approach shows a subtle area of heterogeneous echogenicity in the left cerebral peduncle (*arrows*) that is not present on the right (*arrowhead*). (*B*) Magnified axial view of *A* focusing on the brainstem. (*C*) Axial and (*D*) coronal ADC maps show corresponding areas of restricted diffusion (*arrows*). Abnormal areas of restricted diffusion are also noted in the bilateral basal ganglia and internal capsules on *D*. MR image and US demonstrate similar findings, with the MR imaging findings being more extensive and more florid than the US findings.

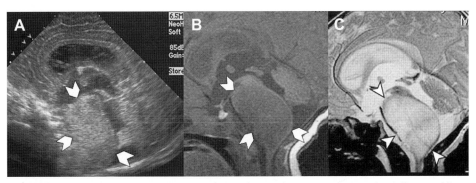

Fig. 14. A 15-day-old, ex-35-week premature infant who underwent a traumatic delivery with persistent nystagmus and seizure activity. (*A*) Sagittal US image shows an echogenic, enlarged pons (*arrowheads*) resulting in mass effect on the 4th ventricle. (*B*) Sagittal T1-weighted image reveals an enlarged, hypointense pons that cannot be clearly differentiated from the medulla or midbrain. (*C*) Sagittal T2-weighted image shows diffuse hyperintensity of the pontine infiltrative lesion (*arrowheads*). Note the hydrocephalus.

because they result in the improved detection of cerebellar injury, compared with when the anterior fontanelle approach alone is used.[49]

Periventricular White Matter

As early as 1984, Siegel and colleagues[33] postulated that increased periventricular echogenicity might be a sign of HII. However, the authors only considered this finding to be positive for HII when it was observed near the external angles of the frontal horns. They used this specification to distinguish HII from the normal halo of increased echogenicity that can be seen in the periatrial white matter because of a sonographic artifact (eg, anisotropism).[50,51] With the use of different

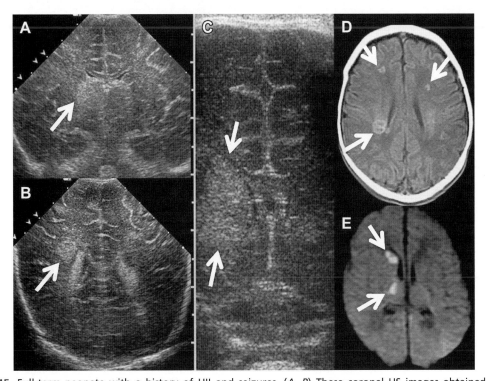

Fig. 15. Full-term neonate with a history of HII and seizures. (*A, B*) These coronal US images obtained with a vector transducer show ill-defined patchy areas of increased echogenicity in the head of the right caudate nucleus and periventricular regions (*arrows*), which are better depicted on the coronal image that was obtained with a linear probe (*arrows* in *C*). (*D*) Axial T1-weighted MR image shows ill-defined rounded foci of hemorrhage in the same areas (*arrows*). (*E*) Axial DWI reveals restricted diffusion in some of these lesions (*arrows*). Although the findings on MR imaging and US are similar, they are more conspicuous on MR imaging.

windows, angled views, and linear transducers, the inability to distinguish HII from the normal area of increased periventricular echogenicity can be easily overcome. The number of different types of abnormalities that can be observed is vast and ranges from subtle focal areas of abnormally increased echogenicity (**Figs. 15** and **16**) to severe PVL (**Fig. 17**). In some cases, a periventricular band of increased echogenicity may be observed, and it may be so dense that it may be difficult to differentiate from periventricular calcifications caused by congenital infections, because the latter rarely display posterior acoustic shadowing in the early neonatal period. This finding is found particularly often in patients with increased ventricular size and transependymal cerebrospinal fluid flow.[52]

Ventricular Size

It is important to recall that even though HII is classically associated with small or slit-like ventricles,

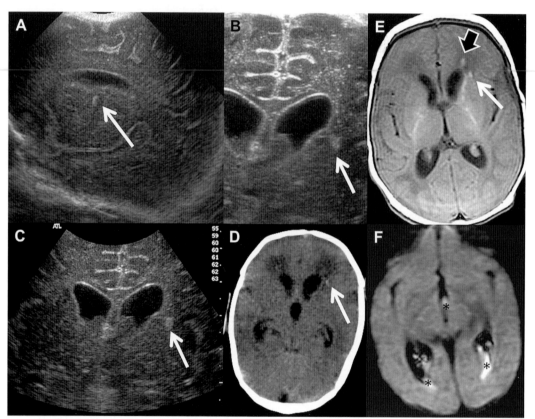

Fig. 16. A 2-week-old infant with seizures, right limb flaccidity, and hypertonicity who was transferred from an outside institution. By report, lumbar puncture revealed findings suggestive of meningitis. (*A*) Sagittal US image shows diffuse accentuation of the GWMD. A small periventricular focus of abnormally increased echogenicity is suggested (*arrow*). (*B*) A coronal magnified US image obtained with a linear transducer and (*C*) a coronal magnified view show abnormally increased echogenicity of the ependymal lining and echogenic material within the frontal horns and the visualized portion of the third ventricle. This may reflect resolving hemorrhage (ie, residual blood products) or, in this clinical scenario, infected debris. The echogenic focus (*arrow*) is better depicted than on *A*, and given the appearance on *D* and *E*, likely reflects a small focus of hemorrhage. (*D*) Unenhanced axial CT image shows a punctate focus of hemorrhage adjacent to the left frontal horn (*arrow*). Edema is noted in both frontal areas. (*E*) Axial T1-weighted image shows a few foci of T1 shortening consistent with the presence of blood products (*white arrow*). The focus indicated with the *black arrow* was not clearly depicted on US. Abnormal signal is also noted along the internal capsules. (*F*) Axial DWI demonstrates increased signal intensity within portions of the occipital horns of both lateral ventricles and in the anterior recess of the third ventricle (*asterisks*). However, no restricted diffusion is noted in the parenchyma, which might be caused by the delay in obtaining the MR image and therefore missing the narrow window of opportunity to image these neonates. Nonetheless, the MR image reveals more extensive injury than US. The US findings are like the "tip of the iceberg" and should trigger MR imaging evaluation to adequately delineate the extent of disease.

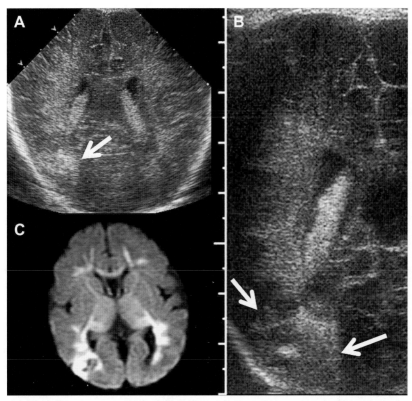

Fig. 17. A 3-day-old, ex-35-week premature infant who underwent a traumatic delivery with persistent seizure activity. (*A*, *B*) Coronal US images show extensive increase in the echogenicity of the periventricular regions bilaterally. In addition, there is a rounded, ill-defined area of more heterogeneous echogenicity in the right peritrigonal area (*arrows*). On MR imaging, this lesion was found to contain blood products and thus was consistent with hemorrhage. (*C*) Axial DWI shows extensive areas of diffusion restriction in the periventricular region consistent with ischemia and reflective of periventricular leukomalacia.

this appearance is only seen in severe cases and only during the first days of life. In the authors' experience, in patients with subtle to moderate brain injury, the ventricular size is usually normal.

DOPPLER US FINDINGS
Resistive Index

The resistive index (RI) is a measure of end organ resistance. It is used to quantify the differences between systolic and diastolic flow velocities (RI = PSV-EDV/PSV). Some authors postulate that the measurement of cerebral blood flow velocities[53] should be preferred to RI measurements, because they consider the former a more accurate indicator of blood flow impairment. However, RI measurements are independent from the angle of insonation that is used and are thus technically more easily to assess. RIs are considered to be normal if they are in the range of 75 ± 10 and they are inversely related to gestational age.[54] Because of the wide range of normal values and because the RI may be affected by

extracranial, particularly cardiac conditions, serial measurements are considered to be more useful in evaluating cerebral blood flow.[55] Decreased RIs (<60[56] or <55[43,57]) during the first 72 hours of life are associated with poor outcomes even in the presence of normal gray-scale findings.[56]

It is recommended that sonographers obtain more than one recording during an ultrasonographic evaluation and even check for variability in the RIs or in the cerebral blood flow velocities over 1 minute or during different times in the study, because it seems that extreme variation occurs in infants with the most severely impaired cerebral autoregulation (**Fig. 18**).[34,36,58]

Hyperemia

It is well known that acute neonatal focal cerebral infarction can lead to an increase in cerebral blood flow to the area. This "luxury cerebral perfusion" is believed to be the result of a loss of neuronal and blood–brain barrier integrity, with secondary release of vasoactive substances and subsequent

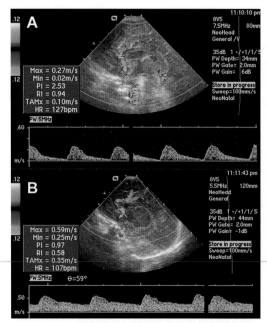

vasodilatation. This increased vascularity can be easily demonstrated on color or power Doppler imaging.[59,60] In the authors' experience, diffuse hyperemia with particular prominence of the lenticulostriate vessels can be demonstrated in cases of severe, profound asphyxia (**Fig. 19**).

Sinus Vein Patency

In the past, sinus vein thrombosis in neonates was often unrecognized; however, because of advancements in imaging techniques, the condition has become increasingly diagnosed in recent times. Interestingly, HII has been established as the most common cause of sinus vein thrombosis in neonates.[61] During the neonatal period, the symptoms are nonspecific and commonly include seizures, jitteriness, and lethargy.[61,62] In many institutions, the superior sagittal sinus is routinely assessed for patency. Sonographic assessment of the normal and the thrombosed superior sagittal sinus has become extremely straightforward since the advent of the use of color Doppler techniques and linear transducers (**Fig. 20**).[38,53] Furthermore, Battin and Teele[63] reported that absent or sluggish flow without evidence of clot formation and followed by the return of normal flow can be detected soon after a hypoxic–ischemic insult occurs.

Fig. 18. A full-term neonate with a history of profound asphyxia. (*A, B*) These spectral display images show RI measurements that were obtained several minutes apart at the level of the anterior cerebral artery and demonstrate marked fluctuation. The variation in these measurements is likely the result of impaired autoregulation.

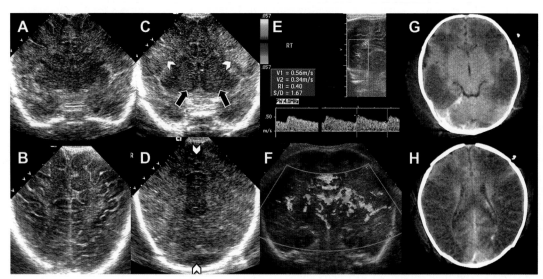

Fig. 19. A 2-week-old full-term neonate with purpura fulminans and severe septic shock. (*A*) Coronal and (*B*) focused coronal US images of the brain periphery show slit-like ventricles and areas of increased GWMD consistent with mild brain edema. (*C, D*) Follow-up US images obtained 2 days later because of the patient's clinical deterioration show interval increase in brain edema with loss of GWMD (*arrowheads* in *C*). There is interval increase in echogenicity of the bilateral basal ganglia (*arrows* in *C*) and blurring of the interhemispheric fissure (*arrowheads* in *D*). (*E*) Doppler evaluation of the anterior cerebral artery reveals an abnormally low resistive index (0.4). (*F*) Coronal color Doppler image shows significant hyperemia in the basal ganglia. (*G, H*) Unenhanced CT images obtained a few hours later show extensive loss of GWMD with sulcal effacement and hypoattenuation involving the frontal, parietal, and occipital lobes (not shown). Extensive scalp edema is also present. This neonate was too sick to be transported to the MR imaging unit and ultimately expired.

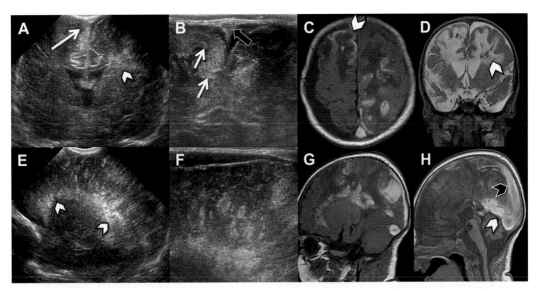

Fig. 20. A 6 week old with congenital heart disease and extensive deep and superficial venous sinus thromboses. (*A*) Coronal US image shows abnormal areas of increased echogenicity in the right frontal region (*arrow*) and the left periventricular white matter (*arrowhead*). (*B*) Coronal US image obtained with a linear transducer better delineates the area noted on *A*, and reflects a thickened, echogenic portion of the cortex (*white arrows*). Note the echogenic material within the visualized portion of the superior sagittal sinus (*black arrow*). On color Doppler imaging (not shown), no flow could be elicited in this region. (*C*) Corresponding axial T1-weighted image reveals cortical laminar necrosis in this area (*arrowhead*). Additional areas of cortical necrosis are seen on the left. (*D*) Coronal T2-weighted image shows similar findings in addition to areas of hemorrhage in the left periventricular area in the distribution of the medullary veins (*arrowhead*). (*E*) Left parasagittal US image shows extensive areas of abnormally increased periventricular echogenicity (*arrowheads*). (*F*) Magnified sagittal view of *E* obtained with a linear transducer better depicts the numerous small fusiform-shaped areas of increased echogenicity. (*G*) Corresponding left parasagittal T1-weighted image demonstrates extensive areas of periventricular hemorrhage in the distribution of the medullary veins. (*H*) Sagittal T1-weighted image shows extensive thrombus formation filling and expanding the straight (*white arrowhead*) and superior sagittal sinus (*black arrowhead*). On MRV (image not shown), sinus vein thrombosis was demonstrated in both the deep and superficial venous systems.

Deep sinus vein thrombosis involving the internal cerebral veins, vein of Galen, or the straight sinus should be suspected in patients in whom cerebral edema or even hemorrhagic lesions are seen in the thalami bilaterally (**Fig. 21**).[62]

DISCUSSION

The described US abnormalities correlate with abnormal MR imaging findings when meticulous attention is paid to the US technique.[34,36] Many of the abnormalities illustrated here represent in essence the "tip of the iceberg" and may point toward the presence of more extensive and florid pathology on MR imaging. However, many of these encephalopathic neonates may be so sick that they cannot be transported to the MR imaging suite. Therefore, recognition of and familiarity with these subtle abnormalities on head US may play an important, complementary role to MR imaging in the evaluation of NE, particularly early in the course of the disease or for follow-up

examinations. In addition, and despite DWI is the ideal imaging technique to use for the evaluation of ischemic lesions, the window of opportunity for its use, unlike in adults, is narrow, because it has previously been shown to be only 1 week postinsult in this age group.[64–66] When imaging is delayed beyond that point, a complete, dedicated US study may potentially help identify the HII-induced changes. MR imaging remains the reference standard for the assessment of ischemic changes, but it is important to remember that MR images should be obtained as early as possible in the course of NE to take advantage of the DWI sequence.[36] Although MR imaging, especially DWI, is the best imaging modality for delineating ischemic changes, the use of daily, repeated, or urgent head US can be extremely effective in patients with NE, especially those who are too sick to be transported to the MR imaging suite.

Optimal results can be obtained when real-time images (not just static images) are evaluated, and when high-frequency transducers of variable

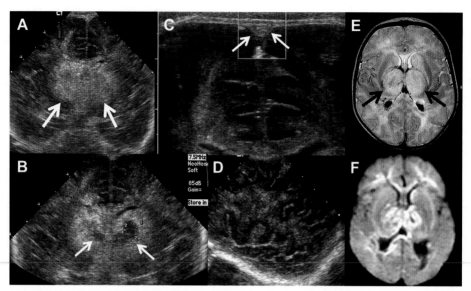

Fig. 21. A 3-week-old, full-term infant, with septic colitis and seizures affecting the left arm. (*A*) Coronal US image shows bilateral areas of abnormally increased echogenicity involving the thalami (*arrows*). (*B*) A magnified focus view of the basal ganglia reveals a more heterogeneous appearance than that noted on *A* with some hypoechogenic regions, likely reflecting evolving hemorrhage (*arrows*). (*C*) Coronal Doppler US image obtained with a linear transducer demonstrates absent flow within the superior sagittal sinus (*arrows*), which is consistent with superior sagittal sinus vein thrombosis. (*D*) Focused US image of the brain periphery demonstrates accentuation of the GWMD consistent with edema. (*E*) Axial T2-weighted image reveals extensive edema in the bilateral thalami (*arrows*), periventricular white matter, and both frontal regions. The same areas demonstrate restricted diffusion on DWI (*F*). These findings are characteristic of deep cerebral venous thrombosis involving the bilateral thalamoperforating veins and bilateral internal cerebral veins. On MRV (image not shown), no flow could be observed in either the superficial or deep venous systems.

configuration, especially the linear array transducers, are used. The use of multiple windows and focused views, especially angled views that include the periphery of the brain, and the use of Doppler analysis including spectral, color, and power are also important in obtaining the most accurate and complete head US results.[34,36]

Historically, head US has been extensively used in the diagnosis and follow-up of newborns in neonatal intensive care units, and the importance of its role has been repeatedly verified by prolonged patient survival rates and improvements in patient outcomes. In recent years, concerns have been raised regarding the use and reliability of head US compared with brain MR imaging.[67–70] This theory is not well supported by studies in which both modalities were compared and particular attention to technique regarding image acquisition and analysis was made.[4,34,36] Although it is well known that US is operator-dependant, currently with up-to-date equipment, use of multiple windows and probes, improved resolution, and the detailed findings one can appreciate on US the use of this modality should not be underestimated. Its role seems to be complementary to MR imaging and it can be used as

a useful adjunct. Furthermore, three-dimensional equipment[71] in development will allow pediatric radiologists to obtain views in any plane. Technical limitations of US and complaints related to anisotropy, poor image quality, or incompleteness of US examinations are likely to decrease, thereby discrediting many US critics. Three-dimensional volume US offers several advantages over two-dimensional imaging. For example, a volumetric acquisition can be stored and reviewed offline. Additionally, multiplanar navigation through the US volume can be pursued, enabling reconstructions in any desired plane to be rendered. Postprocessing filters can also be used to improve tissue contrast and remove artifact. The only argument that may remain against the use of US is interobserver variability.[72,73] Considering costs and availability, and lack of radiation and sedation, investment in development and expansion of US is warranted. Some authors have recommended the implementation of more widespread, formal training in US scanning techniques, neuroanatomy, neurodevelopment, and neuropathology, with formal evaluations of these skills and competencies.[4,43] However, in the authors' experience, such simple steps as increased collaboration between neonatologists, neuroradiologists, sonographers, and pediatric radiologists in the form of weekly or more frequent rounds may significantly improve the quality of the examinations and the interpretation of head US.

SUMMARY

With the implementation of these meticulous practices and techniques the reliability of head US to depict NE changes will improve. The authors strongly recommend the implementation of regular formal meetings between sonographers, pediatric radiologists, neuroradiologists, and neonatologists to improve the use of these studies.

REFERENCES

1. Ferriero DM. Neonatal brain injury. N Engl J Med 2004;351(19):1985–95.
2. Sarnat HB, Sarnat MS. Neonatal encephalopathy following fetal distress: a clinical and electroencephalographic study. Arch Neurol 1976;33(10):696–705.
3. Neufeld MD, Frigon C, Graham AS, et al. Maternal infection and risk of cerebral palsy in term and preterm infants. J Perinatol 2004;25(2):108–13.
4. de Vries LS, Cowan FM. Evolving understanding of hypoxic-ischemic encephalopathy in the term infant. Semin Pediatr Neurol 2009;16(4):216–25.
5. Leijser LM, Steggerda SJ, de Bruïne FT, et al. Lenticulostriate vasculopathy in very preterm infants. Arch Dis Child Fetal Neonatal Ed 2010;95(1):F42–6.
6. Perlman JM. Intrapartum asphyxia and cerebral palsy: is there a link? Clin Perinatol 2006;33(2):335–53.
7. Shah P, Riphagen S, Beyene J, et al. Multiorgan dysfunction in infants with post-asphyxial hypoxic-ischaemic encephalopathy. Arch Dis Child Fetal Neonatal Ed 2004;89(2):F152–5.
8. Martin-Ancel A, Garcia-Alix A, Gaya F, et al. Multiple organ involvement in perinatal asphyxia. J Pediatr 1995;127(5):786–93.
9. Hankins GD, Speer M. Defining the pathogenesis and pathophysiology of neonatal encephalopathy and cerebral palsy. Obstet Gynecol 2003;102(3):628–36.
10. Speer M, Hankins GD. Defining the true pathogenesis and pathophysiology of neonatal encephalopathy and cerebral palsy. J Perinatol 2003;23(3):179–80.
11. Hankins GD. The long journey: defining the true pathogenesis and pathophysiology of neonatal encephalopathy and cerebral palsy. Obstet Gynecol Surv 2003;58(7):435–7.
12. MacLennan A. A template for defining a causal relation between acute intrapartum events and cerebral palsy: international consensus statement. BMJ 1999;319(7216):1054–9.
13. Badawi N, Kurinczuk JJ, Keogh JM, et al. Antepartum risk factors for newborn encephalopathy: the Western Australian case-control study. BMJ 1998;317(7172):1549–53.
14. Badawi N, Kurinczuk JJ, Keogh JM, et al. Intrapartum risk factors for newborn encephalopathy: the Western Australian case-control study. BMJ 1998;317(7172):1554–8.
15. Cowan F, Rutherford M, Groenendaal F, et al. Origin and timing of brain lesions in term infants with neonatal encephalopathy. Lancet 2003;361(9359):736–42.
16. Bax M, Tydeman C, Flodmark O. Clinical and MRI correlates of cerebral palsy: the European Cerebral Palsy Study. JAMA 2006;296(13):1602–8.
17. Graham EM, Ruis KA, Hartman AL, et al. A systematic review of the role of intrapartum hypoxia-ischemia in the causation of neonatal encephalopathy. Am J Obstet Gynecol 2008;199(6):587–95.
18. Nelson KB. Preventing cerebral palsy: paths not (yet) taken. Dev Med Child Neurol 2009;51(10):765–6.
19. Nelson KB. Infection in pregnancy and cerebral palsy. Dev Med Child Neurol 2009;51(4):253–4.
20. Miller SP, Latal B, Clark H, et al. Clinical signs predict 30-month neurodevelopmental outcome after neonatal encephalopathy. Am J Obstet Gynecol 2004;190(1):93–9.
21. Thompson C, Puterman A, Linley L, et al. The value of a scoring system for hypoxic ischaemic encephalopathy in predicting neurodevelopmental outcome. Acta Paediatr 1997;86(7):757–61.
22. Volpe JJ. Neurology of the newborn. 4th edition. Philadelphia: W.B. Saunders; 2001.
23. Berger R, Garnier Y. Perinatal brain injury. J Perinat Med 2000;28(4):261–85.
24. Rutherford MA. MRI of the neonatal brain. Philadelphia: WB Saunders; 2002.
25. Barkovich AJ, Truwit CL. Brain damage from perinatal asphyxia: correlation of MR findings with gestational age. AJNR Am J Neuroradiol 1990;11(6):1087–96.
26. Barkovich AJ. Pediatric neuroimaging. 4th edition. Philadelphia: Lippincott Williams & Wilkins; 2005.
27. Blumenthal I. Periventricular leucomalacia: a review. Eur J Pediatr 2004;163(8):435–42.
28. Volpe JJ. Neonatal periventricular hemorrhage: past, present, and future. J Pediatr 1978;92(4):693–6.
29. Fellman V, Raivio KO. Reperfusion injury as the mechanism of brain damage after perinatal asphyxia. Pediatr Res 1997;41(5):599–606.
30. Kendall G, Peebles D. Acute fetal hypoxia: the modulating effect of infection. Early Hum Dev 2005;81(1):27–34.
31. Martin DJ, Hill A, Fitz CR, et al. Hypoxic/ischaemic cerebral injury in the neonatal brain. A report of

sonographic features with computed tomographic correlation. Pediatr Radiol 1983;13(6):307–12.

32. Babcock DS, Ball W Jr. Postasphyxial encephalopathy in full-term infants: ultrasound diagnosis. Radiology 1983;148(2):417–23.

33. Siegel MJ, Shackelford GD, Perlman JM, et al. Hypoxic-ischemic encephalopathy in term infants: diagnosis and prognosis evaluated by ultrasound. Radiology 1984;152(2):395–9.

34. Daneman A, Epelman M, Blaser S, et al. Imaging of the brain in full-term neonates: does sonography still play a role? Pediatr Radiol 2006;36(7):636–46.

35. Eken P, Jansen GH, Groenendaal F, et al. Intracranial lesions in the fullterm infant with hypoxic ischaemic encephalopathy: ultrasound and autopsy correlation. Neuropediatrics 2010;25(6):301–7.

36. Epelman MD, Daneman A, Kellenberger CJ, et al. Neonatal encephalopathy: a prospective comparison of head US and MRI. Pediatr Radiol 2010; 40(10):1640–50.

37. Winkler P. Advances in paediatric CNS ultrasound. Eur J Radiol 1998;26(2):109–20.

38. Thomson GD, Teele RL. High-frequency linear array transducers for neonatal cerebral sonography. AJR Am J Roentgenol 2001;176(4):995–1001.

39. Breitbach-Faller N, Schrader K, Rating D, et al. Ultrasound findings in follow-up investigations in a case of aspartoacylase deficiency (Canavan disease). Neuropediatrics 2003;34(2):96–9.

40. Harbord MG, LeQuesne GW. Alexander's disease: cranial ultrasound findings. Pediatr Radiol 1988; 18(3):227–8.

41. Connolly B, Kelehan P, O'Brien N, et al. The echogenic thalamus in hypoxic ischaemic encephalopathy. Pediatr Radiol 1994;24(4):268–71.

42. Soghier LM, Vega M, Aref K, et al. Diffuse basal ganglia or thalamus hyperechogenicity in preterm infants. J Perinatol 2006;26(4):230–6.

43. Leijser LM, de Vries LS, Cowan FM. Using cerebral ultrasound effectively in the newborn infant. Early Hum Dev 2006;82(12):827–35.

44. Schlesinger AE, Munden MM, Hayman LA. Hyperechoic foci in the thalamic region imaged via the posterior fontanelle: a potential mimic of thalamic pathology. Pediatr Radiol 1999;29(7):520–3.

45. Di Salvo DN. A new view of the neonatal brain: clinical utility of supplemental neurologic US imaging windows. Radiographics 2001;21(4):943–55.

46. Kock C, Helmke K, Winkler P. The region of the midbrain. Anatomy and peculiarities of its presentation in sonography. Anat Clin 1985;7(3):209–14.

47. Helmke K, Winkler P, Kock C. Sonographic examination of the brain stem area in infants. An echographic and anatomic analysis. Pediatr Radiol 1987;17(1):1–6.

48. Schomerus L, Merkenschlager A, Kahn T, et al. Spontaneous remission of a diffuse brainstem lesion in a neonate. Pediatr Radiol 2007;37(4):399–402.

49. Steggerda SJ, Leijser LM, Wiggers-de Bruïne FT, et al. Cerebellar injury in preterm infants: incidence and findings on US and MR images. Radiology 2009;252(1):190–9.

50. Slovis TL, Shankaran S. Ultrasound in the evaluation of hypoxic-ischemic injury and intracranial hemorrhage in neonates: the state of the art. Pediatr Radiol 1984;14(2):67–75.

51. Guillerman RP. Infant craniospinal ultrasonography: beyond hemorrhage and hydrocephalus. Semin Ultrasound CT MR 2010;31(2):71–85.

52. Daneman A, Lobo E, Mosskin M. Periventricular band of increased echogenicity: edema or calcification? Pediatr Radiol 1998;28(2):83–5.

53. Couture A, Veyrac C, Baud C, et al. Advanced cranial ultrasound: transfontanellar Doppler imaging in neonates. Eur Radiol 2001;11(12):2399–410.

54. Seibert JJ, McCowan TC, Chadduck WM, et al. Duplex pulsed Doppler US versus intracranial pressure in the neonate: clinical and experimental studies. Radiology 1989;171(1):155–9.

55. Bulas DI, Vezina GL. Preterm anoxic injury. Radiologic evaluation. Radiol Clin North Am 1999;37(6): 1147–61.

56. Stark JE, Seibert JJ. Cerebral artery Doppler ultrasonography for prediction of outcome after perinatal asphyxia. J Ultrasound Med 1994;13(8):595–600.

57. Archer LN, Levene MI, Evans DH. Cerebral artery Doppler ultrasonography for prediction of outcome after perinatal asphyxia. Lancet 1986;2(8516): 1116–8.

58. Coughtrey H, Rennie JM, Evans DH. Variability in cerebral blood flow velocity: observations over one minute in preterm babies. Early Hum Dev 1997; 47(1):63–70.

59. Taylor GA. Alterations in regional cerebral blood flow in neonatal stroke: preliminary findings with color Doppler sonography. Pediatr Radiol 1994;24(2): 111–5.

60. Steventon DM, John PR. Power Doppler ultrasound appearances of neonatal ischaemic brain injury. Pediatr Radiol 1997;27(2):147–9.

61. deVeber G, Andrew M, Adams C, et al. Cerebral sinovenous thrombosis in children. N Engl J Med 2001;345(6):417–23.

62. Shroff M, deVeber G. Sinovenous thrombosis in children. Neuroimaging Clin N Am 2003;13(1):115–38.

63. Battin MR, Teele RL. Abnormal sagittal sinus blood flow in term infants following a perinatal hypoxic ischaemic insult. Pediatr Radiol 2003;33(8):559–62.

64. Melhem ER. Time-course of apparent diffusion coefficient in neonatal brain injury: the first piece of the puzzle. Neurology 2002;59(6):798–9.

65. Mader I, Schoning M, Klose U, et al. Neonatal cerebral infarction diagnosed by diffusion-weighted MRI: pseudonormalization occurs early. Stroke 2002; 33(4):1142–5.

66. Winter JD, Lee DS, Hung RM, et al. Apparent diffusion coefficient pseudonormalization time in neonatal hypoxic-ischemic encephalopathy. Pediatr Neurol 2007;37(4):255–62.

67. Woodward LJ, Anderson PJ, Austin NC, et al. Neonatal MRI to predict neurodevelopmental outcomes in preterm infants. N Engl J Med 2006;355(7):685–94.

68. Debillon T, N'Guyen S, Muet A, et al. Limitations of ultrasonography for diagnosing white matter damage in preterm infants. Arch Dis Child Fetal Neonatal Ed 2003;88(4):F275–9.

69. Mirmiran M, Barnes PD, Keller K, et al. Neonatal brain magnetic resonance imaging before discharge is better than serial cranial ultrasound in predicting cerebral palsy in very low birth weight preterm infants. Pediatrics 2004;114(4):992–8.

70. Childs AM, Cornette L, Ramenghi LA, et al. Magnetic resonance and cranial ultrasound characteristics of periventricular white matter abnormalities in newborn infants. Clin Radiol 2001;56(8):647–55.

71. Vinals F, Munoz M, Naveas R, et al. Transfrontal three-dimensional visualization of midline cerebral structures. Ultrasound Obstet Gynecol 2007;30(2):162–8.

72. Harris DL, Bloomfield FH, Teele RL, et al. Variable interpretation of ultrasonograms may contribute to variation in the reported incidence of white matter damage between newborn intensive care units in New Zealand. Arch Dis Child Fetal Neonatal Ed 2006;91(1):F11–6.

73. Kuban K, Adler I, Allred EN, et al. Observer variability assessing US scans of the preterm brain: the ELGAN study. Pediatr Radiol 2007;37(12):1201–8.

MR Imaging-Guided Cardiovascular Interventions in Young Children

Aphrodite Tzifa, MD, MRCPCH[a,c,*], Tobias Schaeffter, PhD[b],
Reza Razavi, MD, FRCP[b,c]

KEYWORDS

- Congenital heart disease • Cardiac catheterization
- MR imaging • Cardiac

Congenital heart disease occurs in 0.8% to 1% of children. Some of these patients will require interventional treatment in the form of cardiac catheterization or surgery, whereas others will require only medical therapy. Echocardiography is the investigation of choice for diagnosis and follow-up of these patients, whereas MR imaging is now increasingly used in most centers to assess complex congenital cases and to answer specific questions, which are not possible to address with echocardiography. The ability to obtain anatomic along with quantitative physiologic information, such as cardiac function and flows, in one examination has led to more detailed assessment and analysis of congenital heart defects. This continues to improve our understanding about congenital heart disease and its treatment options.

Cardiac catheterization procedures, routinely performed up to a few years ago to aid diagnosis, have now been mostly replaced by cardiac MR imaging scans. In parallel, a new form of hybrid catheterization has emerged that combines MR imaging with simultaneous pressure measurement in different cardiac chambers and vascular structures. The combination of radiographic (ie, x-ray) and MR imaging (XMR)-guided catheterizations can accurately address clinical questions, such as estimation of pulmonary vascular resistance (PVR) and cardiac output response to stress, without the limitation of hemodynamic assumptions during calculations.[1–8] Also, for more accurate physiologic information, XMR catheterization can also offer detailed anatomic information of structures not well seen on echocardiography or MR imaging alone, such as small aortopulmonary collateral arteries, so that fluoroscopy and MR imaging can be combined in one procedure to avoid two general-anesthetic sessions in the same child and for the same purpose.

Beyond diagnosis, MR imaging currently expands its potential by guiding interventional procedures that may be performed in the MR imaging scanner in a similar fashion and with similar equipment to the ones used in the traditional

Funding sources: This work was supported by the UK Department of Health via the National Institute for Health Research (NIHR) comprehensive Biomedical Research Centre award to Guy's & St Thomas' NHS Foundation Trust in partnership with King's College London (AT).
Disclosures: The investigators received research grant support from Philips Healthcare.
^a Division of Imaging Sciences, King's College London BHF Centre, NIHR Biomedical Research Centre at Guy's & St Thomas' Hospital NHS Foundation Trust, Westminster Bridge Road, London SE1 7EH, UK
^b Division of Imaging Sciences, King's College London BHF Centre, Rayne Institute, St Thomas' Hospital, Guy's & St Thomas' Hospital Trust, Westminster Bridge Road, London SE1 7EH, UK
^c Department of Paediatric Cardiology, Evelina Children's Hospital, Guy's & St Thomas' Hospital NHS Trust, Westminster Bridge Road, London SE1 7EH, UK
* Corresponding author.
E-mail address: aphrodite.tzifa@kcl.ac.uk

Magn Reson Imaging Clin N Am 20 (2012) 117–128
doi:10.1016/j.mric.2011.08.011

catheterization suite. This article discusses in detail how MR imaging can be used for interventional diagnosis and treatment in young children with congenital heart disease.

MR IMAGING-GUIDED DIAGNOSTIC CARDIAC CATHETERIZATIONS
MR Imaging-Guided Diagnostic Catheterizations Combined with Radiographic Imaging

In the current era, diagnostic cardiac catheterizations have been greatly replaced either by MR imaging scans or by XMR catheterizations. The latter have been shown to entail lower radiation exposure doses when compared with controls,[2] which is of particular importance in children with congenital heart disease who are usually subjected to various and repetitive procedures involving radiation. According to the UK National Radiation Protection Board, the mean risk of solid tumor development as a result of a single cardiac catheterization procedure is approximately 1 in 2500 in adults. This risk increases to 1 in 1000 in children if exposure occurs by the age of 5 years.[9] Also, the proportion of the body that is irradiated increases as the size of the patient decreases, which, coupled with the increased radiosensitivity of the young and immature tissues, explains recent evidence showing that these children are at higher risk of developing cancer in later life.[10–12]

A further benefit of XMR-guided catheterizations is the improved soft tissue characterization and visualization of cardiac structures and vessels, in contrast to radiographic-guided catheterizations, which rely on identification of landmarks and contrast angiography. XMR catheterizations also provide physiologic data, that are not possible to obtain during radiographic catheterization and that are essential for the assessment of complex patients. Such data involve cardiac output assessment, estimation of the pulmonary to systemic flow ratio (Qp/Qs), flows and maximum velocities across valves and in large vessels, pressure-volume loop relationships, and ventricular function.[13–19] In addition, PVR and compliance can be accurately assessed using invasive pressure measurements and magnetic resonance (MR) flow data.[20–23]

Equipment
XMR catheterizations take place in specifically designed catheterization laboratories with combined radiographic and MR imaging facilities (**Fig. 1**). In the authors' laboratory, a 1.5T MR imaging scanner (Achieva, Philips, Best, Netherlands) and a Philips BV Pulsera cardiac radiographic unit are used. There are in-room monitor and controls, which

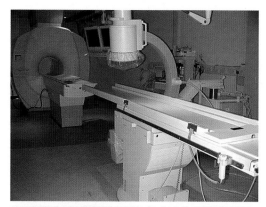

Fig. 1. The XMR interventional suite at King's College (Guy's Hospital Campus), London, UK, is comprised of a 1.5 T MR imaging scanner (Achieva Philips, Best, Netherlands) and a single plane mobile cardiac radiographic set (Philips BV Pulsera). Patients can be moved in less than 60 sec between the two systems using a specially modified sliding table. The ceiling-mounted MR imaging monitor and controls are positioned next to the magnet.

can swing across the bottom end and the top end of the magnet, and display MR images and hemodynamic pressure traces (**Fig. 2**). The fluoroscopic area and MR field of an XMR laboratory can be separated either by doors or by a clearly defined line, demarcating the 5-gauss line of the magnet, beyond which it is possible for electronic devices, such as echocardiography machines and computer equipment, to be brought into the room (**Fig. 3**). The tabletop design allows patients to be moved from one modality to the other in a very short time. Furthermore, the table position is stored within the system allowing image fusion between the MR imaging and radiographic system (ie, XMR) or

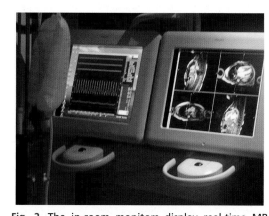

Fig. 2. The in-room monitors display real-time MR images and hemodynamic pressure traces during the MR imaging-guided intervention. They can be moved across the bottom end and the top end of the magnet to be in proximity to the interventional cardiologist.

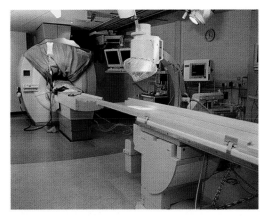

Fig. 3. A second drape is taped to the top of the magnet to ensure sterility inside the MR imaging scanner.

even fusion with other imaging modalities (eg, echocardiography).[24]

After the patient is placed on the table in the nonmagnetic area of the XMR room, the MR imaging coil and ECG leads are placed. MR-compatible patient monitoring and anesthetic equipment is used. For pressure monitoring, we use the commercially available hemodynamic monitoring system EP Tracer 102 (CardioTek B.V, Maastricht, the Netherlands). All of the anesthetic and monitoring tubing and lines are designed with extra length and are secured to the movable tabletop to ensure smooth patient transfer. The ECG and invasive pressure data are sent from the MR-compatible monitoring equipment via an optical network to a computer in the control room where the cardiac technician is stationed. The appropriate measurement and recording of the data is made in the usual way. The technician has access to monitors that show the appropriate radiographs or MR images of the procedure. Blood samples taken during the procedure are labeled in the room and passed to the technician in the control room. Monitoring of the cardiac rhythm during XMR catheterization is achieved with a vector electrocardiogram (VCG). The QRS detection algorithm automatically adjusts to the actual electrical axis of the patient's heart and the specific multidimensional QRS waveform. This greatly improves the reliability of R wave detection to nearly 100%. A reliable R wave, with the P and T waves that are also always clearly seen with VCG, allows detection of nearly all arrhythmias. Unfortunately, there are no ECG systems that can reliably provide ST segment or T wave morphologic information. In the future, using signal-processing techniques may make it possible to improve ECG monitoring during MR imaging scanning.

Significant consideration has been given in the design, construction, and operation of the authors' XMR facility with regard to safety, and a comprehensive safety protocol has been drawn up in our laboratory to minimize possible hazards (**Box 1**).

XMR catheterization procedure

The children are prepared in a similar fashion to those undergoing routine cardiac catheterization. In the authors' department, the patients are anesthetized and recovered in a dedicated area adjacent to the MR imaging scanning area. They are wheeled into the MR imaging room on MR-compatible trolleys and the procedure starts with cardiac catheterization in the nonmagnetic field area of the XMR laboratory. The facilities and equipment of the x-ray area are similar to the traditional catheterization laboratory. A non–MR-compatible angiographic pump is brought into the laboratory and used for detailed angiography, when needed. Standard ECG leads are placed along with a three-lead ECG attached to the anesthetic machine and the VCG, to use for cardiac monitoring during MR imaging scanning. The VCG electrodes are placed on the subcostal margin, outside the radiographic field of view, and the VCG is used for triggering MR imaging

Box 1
XMR facility: safety features
Compulsory safety training of all MR imaging interventional staff
Specially designed clothes without pockets
Safety officer restricting entry to the main room during XMR intervention
Clear demarcation of ferromagnetic safe and unsafe areas within the room
MR-compatible anesthetic and monitoring equipment
Noise-proof headphone systems for all staff within the room
Scrub room shielded from x-rays and radiofrequencies
Positive-pressure air handling and filtration system
Tethering of all ferromagnetic equipment to the wall or floor
Safety checks whenever a patient is transferred between x-ray and MR areas to ensure that metallic instruments used for catheterization are not taken across to the MR end of the room
Written log of all safety infringements and regular review of safety procedures

scans. An MR-compatible pulse oximeter and noninvasive blood pressure monitoring equipment are also attached. The exhaled anesthetic gases are monitored for end-tidal carbon dioxide and for the concentration of the volatile anesthetic agents. Flexible phased array radiofrequency (RF) coils are used. These coils are relatively x-ray lucent and do not need to be removed between radiographic and MR imaging.

After femoral venous and arterial access is obtained, a heparin bolus of 50 IU/kg is given with activated clotting time (ACT) monitoring. After right and/or left heart catheterization is completed under x-ray guidance, the patient is moved across to the MR imaging scanner on the sliding table after the standard ECG leads are removed and safety checks have been performed. These include an operating theater-style check of all metallic objects used under x-ray. Once the patient is inside the scanner, a second drape is placed and then lifted up and taped to the top of the magnet, which, in effect, provides sterile draping of the bore and sides of the magnet (see **Fig. 3**). MR-compatible catheters (Wedge Catheter, Arrow, Reading, PA, USA) placed during fluoroscopic-guided cardiac catheterization are left in situ, usually in the right ventricle or main pulmonary artery (MPA) for continuous hemodynamic pressure monitoring. Invasive arterial pressure is monitored through a femoral arterial cannula or sheath. Simultaneous MR imaging phase contrast or MR cine scans and pressure recording are performed. These give the physician a "snapshot" of the patient's physiology at that particular time and reflect the conditions that they may have been subjected to (ie, nitric oxide administration during PVR assessment or dobutamine stress testing). In addition, a free-breathing, ECG-triggered, three-dimensional (3D) steady state free precession (SSFP) scan of the heart and great vessels and a 3D contrast-enhanced MR angiography are also performed to elucidate intracardiac and vascular anatomy.

The authors have performed more than 160 cardiac catheterizations for congenital heart disease in their XMR laboratory. Some of these have involved combined x-ray and MR-guided procedures, whereas others have been performed solely under MR guidance. Most of the catheterization procedures were performed for PVR measurement, although several were performed to define anatomy, perform XMR-guided interventions (**Fig. 4**), or assess the cardiac stress response to dobutamine.

Assessment of pulmonary vascular resistance PVR studies have been performed either with fluoroscopic or MR guidance. There is no patient age limit for the performance of these studies, but

higher spatial resolution is required for phase contrast flow imaging in infants to ensure there are enough pixels covering the vessel of interest for accurate flow measurements. With the technique described above, the patient undergoes an MR imaging scan and phase contrast flow images are obtained in the MPA, right pulmonary artery (RPA), left pulmonary artery (LPA), and aorta with simultaneous pressure monitoring. For patients with univentricular heart palliation, flows will be assessed in the branch pulmonary arteries for PVR estimation, and in the two caval veins, the neoaorta (and native aorta, when of good size) for detailed assessment of the physiology and the flow distribution.

When the PVR at baseline is raised, 100% fraction of inspired oxygen and nitric oxide 20 ppm are given and the PVR is recalculated. It is important to obtain oxygen saturation and a blood gas at the beginning of the procedure and during different stages of the protocol, as dictated by the patient's clinical condition and end-tidal carbon dioxide. This is to ensure a steady anesthetic state and normocarbia, which is vital for accurate PVR measurement because the latter can swing and be inadvertently elevated if the carbon dioxide levels are allowed to rise. The authors have found moderate to good agreement between the Fick method and the MR method of deriving PVR at baseline conditions.[2] However, in the presence of nitric oxide, which is used to assess pulmonary vasoreactivity, there was less agreement between the two methods. There was not only worsening in agreement but also a large bias when PVR was measured in the presence of 100% oxygen and nitric oxide. We believe that this is the result of errors in the Fick method rather than the XMR method, which has important implications for patient management, particularly of young children. To this end, we suggest that PVR measurement in children is performed with the MR method wherever possible.

Dobutamine stress study for assessment of cardiac output response Dobutamine stress study for assessment of the cardiac output response is regularly required in young infants and children, such as children with Alagille syndrome and pulmonary artery stenosis or, more rarely, in children with univentricular heart circulation. MR imaging is the ideal tool for the evaluation of cardiac function and cardiac output. When combined with dobutamine stress it allows the measurement of right and left ventricular function, cardiac output, and cardiac output in response to stress and systemic vasodilation.

Adding to a full anatomic assessment, MR imaging cardiac catheterization combined with

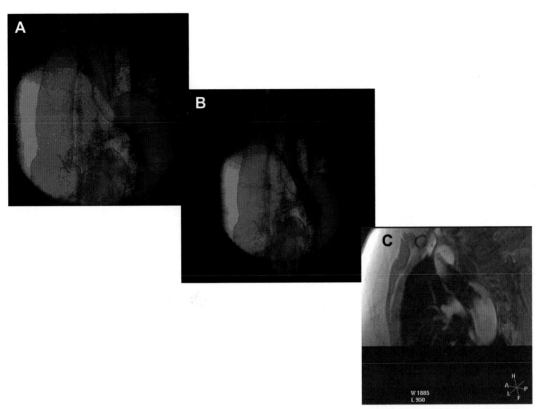

Fig. 4. Aortic stent implantation using XMR-guidance system. An MR angiography image is superimposed onto the fluoroscopic image during stent implantation for native aortic coarctation with very tortuous aortic arch (*A*). A bespoke made covered Cheatham-platinum stent was implanted across the coarctation in the x-ray part of the XMR laboratory (*B*). Following stent implantation the patient was moved back to the scanner and a repeat MR imaging study showed good stent position and no areas of dissection (*C*).

dobutamine stress enables evaluation of the right ventricle (RV) pressure compared with systemic, the RV systolic and diastolic function in response to stress, the gradient across the pulmonary valve or branch pulmonary arteries and the pulmonary artery pressure, and PVR. If the PVR is elevated, pulmonary vasodilators can be administered and the patient's PVR and hemodynamics are reassessed. Selective angiography can also be performed to address clinical questions, such as pulmonary arteriovenous malformations or abnormal collateral vessels that are not clearly visualized on MR imaging.

The authors' MR imaging with dobutamine stress scan protocol is described as follows: We always ensure that the patient is not intravascularly dry because this may affect the cardiac output response to stress. After femoral venous and arterial access is obtained, a heparin bolus of 30 to 50 IU/kg is given with ACT monitoring. Right heart catheterization is performed either with fluoroscopic or MR imaging guidance. Pressure measurements are obtained in the femoral artery, inferior vena cava, right atrium, right ventricle, MPA, LPA (proximal and distal), RPA (proximal and distal), RPA and LPA wedge, or left atrium if an atrial communication is present. An MR imaging compatible catheter (wedge catheter) is left in the RV and an MR imaging scan is performed. This includes a four-chamber view, RV and LV outflow tract views in two planes, Gad MRA, 3D-volume SSFP scan, short axis stack (for LV and RV functional assessment), phase contrast flow images in the aorta and pulmonary artery (for assessment of cardiac output and shunt), and differential branch pulmonary artery flows. The PVR is obtained from a pulmonary artery flow measurement combined with direct pressure measurement, as described above. After baseline data are obtained, dobutamine is infused at 10 μg/kg/min and repeat short axis stack and phase contrast flows in the aorta and pulmonary artery are obtained. The infusion is then increased to 20 μg/kg/min with repeat short axis stack and phase contrast flows in the aorta and pulmonary artery. We aim for a heart rate increase of more than 50% from baseline. After all physiologic measurements have been obtained, the dobutamine infusion is discontinued and the patient is woken up and extubated. Children are observed on the ward for a few hours after anesthetic and are usually discharged home the same day.

Value of dobutamine stress studies in patients before liver transplantation The value of dobutamine stress studies in patients with Alagille syndrome and branch pulmonary artery stenosis has been demonstrated.[25] It was concluded that patients with a maximal increase in cardiac output of less than 40% and/or a right ventricular to aortic pressure ratio of equal or greater than 0.5 should be considered at higher risk and were associated with less favorable outcome following liver transplantation. This study was not performed in an XMR setting, but in the cardiac catheterization laboratory, using a flow-directed thermodilution catheter, and cardiac output calculations were performed on a dedicated computer (Vigalence, Baxter, Newbury, Berkshire, UK). In the current era, MR imaging would easily obtain the above calculations, with assessment of the ventricular function and volumes, as well as flows across the great vessels.

Solely MR Imaging-Guided Diagnostic Cardiac Catheterizations

MR imaging-guided catheterizations have been diagnostic in nature (in humans) and interventional (in animals). Visualization has been aided by passive and active visualization techniques and catheter tracking. Passive tracking technique is commonly based on visualization of susceptibility artifacts or signal voids caused by the interventional device under MR imaging,[26–29] whereas active catheter tracking and visualization uses an electrical connection to the MR imaging scanner, and localization or tracking of the device requires the device itself, along with any additional hardware or software that comes with it. Typically, the device is equipped with a coil or an antenna that functions in either receive-only mode or transmit–receive mode.[30–36]

Active guidewires that have been used for MR imaging-guide interventions in animals are tracked or visualized by employing miniature RF coils or loopless antenna each connected to the scanner using a long metallic wire. This long wire can heat up during certain MR imaging sequences due to resonating RF waves. Despite modifications to reduce the risk of heating with active devices, under certain conditions heating at the tip can occur up to 70°C with obvious associated risks.[37] New strategies for RF-safe active devices have been proposed, including optical transmission and use of transformers to shorten the length of the conducting wire (**Figs. 5** and **6**).[38,39] However, no clinically safe active guidewires have been developed so far. Semiactive catheters use tuned fiducial markers that produce increased MR signal locally without wires connecting to the scanner.[40] There are, however, issues with miniaturization and the ability of firmly securing these markers to catheters.

Passive devices, such as the ones used in the authors' laboratory, have the advantages of having no risk of heating and of lower cost, but the disadvantages of being less visible than active guide wires and requiring manual tracking and changing of the imaging plane to keep the wire in view. To

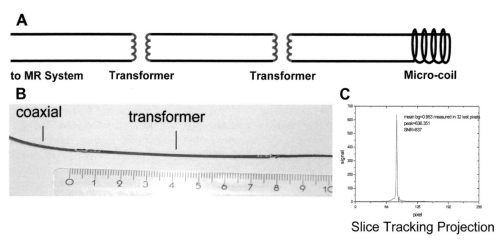

Fig. 5. Concept of the transformer-based cable for RF safety. (*A*) Transformers split a long cable into several short, nonresonant, and, thus, RF-safe sections. (*B*) Miniature transformer (diameter 1 mm) and coax-cable can be integrated into a catheter lumen. (*C*) Tracking signal with high signal-to-noise ratio allows reliable and RF-safe catheter tracking. (*Courtesy of* Steffen Weiss, Philips Research.)

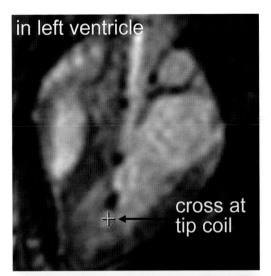

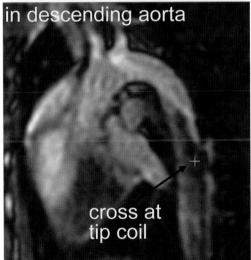

Fig. 6. RF-safe catheter tracking in a pig experiment. The position of the microcoil attached on the catheter tip is measured and displayed (*cross*) on real-time MR images. (*Courtesy of* Steffen Weiss, Philips Research.)

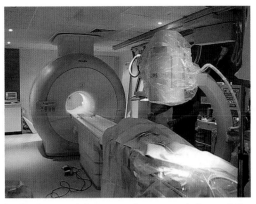

Fig. 7. Foot pedals are used to control the real-time MR imaging interface (eg, to start or stop real-time MR imaging and to change between different predefined geometries).

following views are stored: superior vena cava or inferior vena cava sagittal and coronal, four-chamber, RV outflow tract, anterior wall RV outflow tract (R2) chamber, pulmonary artery bifurcation, LPA sagittal, and RPA coronal views. The patients are placed on the radiograph table, where sheaths are inserted after securing the chosen MR imaging coil and placement of the VCG leads. The patient is then moved into the scanner and the cardiac catheterization is performed under sole MR imaging guidance (**Fig. 9**). The in-room console displays the hemodynamic pressures on one panel and four chosen imaging planes on the other (see **Fig. 2**). An interactive SSFP sequence (8–10 frames/sec) with real-time manipulation of scan parameters is used. The operators can start and stop the MR imaging scan independently with foot pedals and rotate through the four imaging planes displayed. The balloon wedge pressure catheter is inserted into the sheath in the right femoral vein and advanced into the inferior vena cava (**Fig. 10**). For this maneuver, a parasagittal imaging plane, showing the inferior and superior vena cava and the right atrium is used. The balloon of the wedge pressure catheter is visualized as a dark signal void within the surrounding bright blood (see **Fig. 10**). As soon as the right atrium is reached, the imaging plane is interactively changed to show the right atrium and right ventricle from different projections (R2 chamber or 4-chamber view). The tricuspid valve is passed and the balloon wedge pressure catheter is advanced into the right ventricle. The imaging plane is then changed to show the outflow tract and then the MPA. The catheter is advanced into both branch pulmonary arteries and the wedge position for detailed pressure measurements

facilitate better visualization, the operators in our XMR laboratory use foot pedals (**Fig. 7**). With those, the operator can start and stop the interactive scanning independently, and adjust the imaging plane and slice position to get the interventional devices in view. The latter is achieved with the foot pedal function, which rotates through preselected imaging planes and the pedal pull-push action.

At the beginning of any MR imaging-guided catheterization, the likely imaging planes needed for subsequent catheter tracking are stored along with the rest of the MR imaging protocol (**Fig. 8**). For example, for right heart catheterization, the

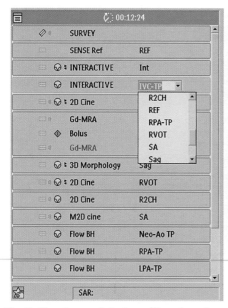

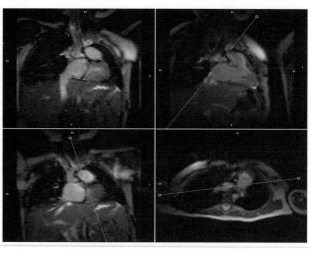

Fig. 8. Planning and storing of imaging planes needed for subsequent visualization of the MR imaging-guided catheterization. Four imaging planes can be put up at the same time for the operator to rotate through during MR imaging-guided catheterization.

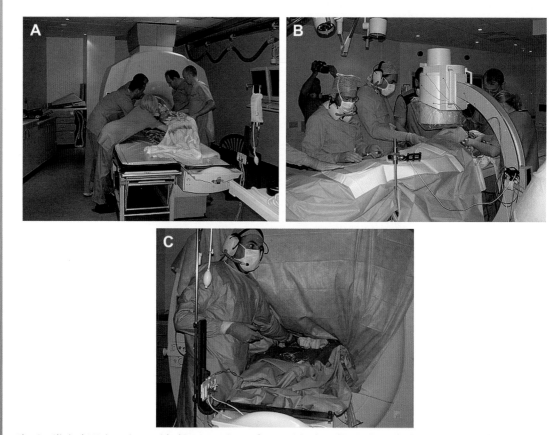

Fig. 9. Clinical MR imaging-guided intervention. After positioning the patient on the XMR table (*A*), the sheaths are inserted outside the MR imaging scanner (*B*). The patient is then moved into the MR imaging magnet and the cardiac catheterization is completely performed under MR imaging guidance (*C*).

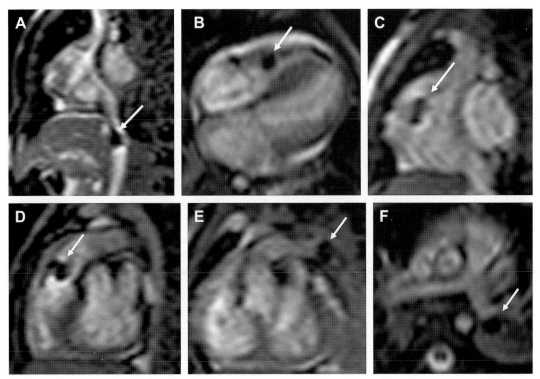

Fig. 10. The balloon of the wedge pressure catheter (*arrows*) is visualized as a dark signal void within the surrounding bright blood in the inferior vena cava (*A*), right ventricle (*B* and *C*), right ventricular outflow tract (*D*), distal LPA in sagittal (*E*), and axial view (*F*).

with pullback gradient recordings as necessary (**Fig. 11**). Because only the tip of the wedge catheter is visualized, care is taken not to push the catheter too fast and, thus, beyond the MR imaging plane. This also ensures that the catheter does not accidentally form loops and possible knots.

For left heart catheterization, the balloon wedge pressure catheter is introduced via the femoral artery, inflated with carbon dioxide and advanced through the descending aorta to the aortic arch. For this step a parasagittal imaging plane is chosen, which shows the aortic arch, the ascending aorta, the aortic valve, and the left ventricle. The balloon of the wedge catheter is visible in the aorta as a signal void. Subsequently, the catheter is turned into the ascending aorta. For this, the use of an MR-compatible guidewire may be necessary because, at this point, the balloon wedge catheter tends to travel up the head and neck vessels instead of down to the ascending aorta. Under MR imaging guidance, it is then possible to cross nonstenotic aortic valves to measure LV pressure. If catheter manipulation into a particular heart chamber or vessel using MR imaging guidance alone is difficult, the patient

is transferred back to the x-ray end of the room where catheterization can be continued under x-ray fluoroscopy (eg, to use a guidewire or a braided catheter). The patient can be transferred back to the MR imaging scanner for further MR measurements once the catheter is positioned satisfactorily.

MR IMAGING-GUIDED INTERVENTIONAL CARDIAC CATHETERIZATIONS

MR imaging-guided interventions had only been performed in animals so far,[41–55] due to the lack of safe and compatible devices for MR imaging, particularly catheters and guidewires. Recently, a compatible and safe guidewire for MR imaging was developed, which has similar characteristics to the guidewires used in the traditional catheterization laboratory. Following a preclinical animal trial to assess the characteristics of this wire, we recently performed the first-in-man, solely MR imaging-guided, interventions in patients with congenital heart disease.[56] The authors currently are running a clinical trial to assess the feasibility, safety, and efficacy of simple percutaneous interventions that involve balloon dilations of stenotic lesions.

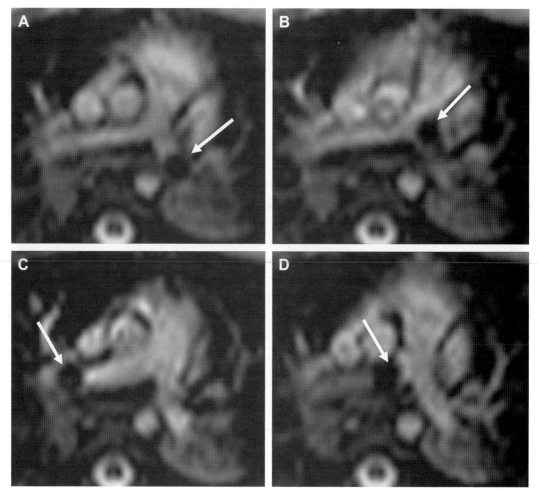

Fig. 11. The balloon wedge catheter (*arrows*) is advanced into both branch pulmonary arteries and pullback gradient recordings are taken as necessary from LPA distal (*A*) to LPA proximal (*B*) and RPA distal (*C*) to RPA proximal (*D*).

However, because the MR imaging-compatible guidewire is 0.035 in and its use is compatible only with bigger balloons (mostly >14 mm); therefore, it is unlikely that these interventions will be applicable to young children of less than 2 years of age.

SUMMARY

Diagnostic cardiac catheterization procedures in children have been largely replaced by MR imaging studies. However, when invasive catheterization is required, MR imaging has a significant role to play. Beyond the established reduction to the radiation dose involved, solely MR image-guided or MR image-assisted catheterization procedures can accurately address clinical questions, such as estimation of PVR and cardiac output response to stress, without needing to perform laborious measurements that are prone to errors. XMR-

guided catheterizations have proven to be valuable and MR imaging-guided interventional cardiac catheterizations show promise for the future.

ACKNOWLEDGMENTS

We are grateful to the members of the pediatric cardiology team of the Evelina Children's Hospital for their support with the care of the pediatric patients that are catheterized in the XMR laboratory and the invaluable help of Shakeel Qureshi, Aaron Bell, Gerald Greil, and Philipp Beerbaum. We would also like to thank Paul James, Dev Mahtani, Shyamala Moganasundram, and other members of the Anesthetic Department involved in interventional MR imaging procedures. Finally, we are very grateful to Rebecca Lund, John Spence, and other members of the Radiology Department for their considerable support and assistance in the performance of these procedures.

REFERENCES

1. Wilkinson JL. Haemodynamic calculations in the catheter laboratory. Heart 2001;85:113–20.
2. Razavi R, Hill DL, Keevil SF, et al. Cardiac catheterisation guided by MRI in children and adults with congenital heart disease. Lancet 2003;362:1877–82.
3. Cigarroa RG, Lange RA, Hillis LD. Oximetric quantitation of intracardiac left-to-right shunting: limitations of the Qp/Qs ratio. Am J Cardiol 1989;64(3):246–7.
4. Dhingra VK, Fenwick JC, Walley KR, et al. Lack of agreement between thermodilution and Fick cardiac output in critically ill patients. Chest 2002;122(3):990–7.
5. Hillis LD, Firth BG, Winniford MD. Variability of right-sided cardiac oxygen saturations in adults with and without left-to-right intracardiac shunting. Am J Cardiol 1986;58(1):129–32.
6. Van den Berg E Jr, Pacifico A, Lange RA, et al. Measurement of cardiac output without right heart catheterization: reliability, advantages, and limitations of a left-sided indicator dilution technique. Cathet Cardiovasc Diagn 1986;12(3):205–8.
7. Hillis LD, Firth BG, Winniford MD. Analysis of factors affecting the variability of Fick versus indicator dilution measurements of cardiac output. Am J Cardiol 1985;56(12):764–8.
8. Dehmer GJ, Firth BG, Hillis LD. Oxygen consumption in adult patients during cardiac catheterization. Clin Cardiol 1982;5(8):436–40.
9. (NRPB) NRPB. Guidelines on patient dose to promote the optimisation of protection for diagnostic medical exposures: report of an advisory group on Ionising. Radiation 1999;10(1).
10. Andreassi MG. Radiation risk from pediatric cardiac catheterisation: friendly fire on children with congenital heart disease. Circulation 2009;120:1847–9.
11. Andreassi MG, Ait-Ali L, Botto N, et al. Cardiac catheterization and long-term chromosomal damage in children with congenital heart disease. Eur Heart J 2006;27:2703–8.
12. Modan B, Keinan L, Blumstein T, et al. Cancer following cardiac catheterization in childhood. Int J Epidemiol 2000;29:424–8.
13. Beerbaum P, Korperich H, Barth P, et al. Noninvasive quantification of left-to-right shunt in pediatric patients: phase-contrast cine magnetic resonance imaging compared with invasive oximetry. Circulation 2001;103(20):2476–82.
14. Beerbaum P, Korperich H, Gieseke J, et al. Rapid left-to-right shunt quantification in children by phase-contrast magnetic resonance imaging combined with sensitivity encoding (SENSE). Circulation 2003;108(11):1355–61.

15. Beerbaum P, Korperich H, Gieseke J, et al. Blood flow quantification in adults by phase-contrast MRI combined with SENSE—a validation study. J Cardiovasc Magn Reson 2005;7(2):361–9.
16. Firmin DN, Nayler GL, Klipstein RH, et al. In vivo validation of MR velocity imaging. J Comput Assist Tomogr 1987;11(5):751–6.
17. Kilner PJ, Manzara CC, Mohiaddin RH, et al. Magnetic resonance jet velocity mapping in mitral and aortic valve stenosis. Circulation 1993;87(4):1239–48.
18. Hundley WG, Li HF, Hillis LD, et al. Quantitation of cardiac output with velocity-encoded, phase difference magnetic resonance imaging. Am J Cardiol 1995;75(17):1250–5.
19. Hundley WG, Li HF, Lange RA, et al. Assessment of left-to-right intracardiac shunting by velocity encoded, phase-difference magnetic resonance imaging. A comparison with oximetric and indicator dilution techniques. Circulation 1995;91(12):2955–60.
20. Mousseaux E, Tasu JP, Jolivet O, et al. Pulmonary arterial resistance: non invasive measurement with indexes of pulmonary flow estimated at velocity-encoded MR imaging–preliminary experience. Radiology 1999;212(3):896–902.
21. Kondo C, Caputo GR, Masui T, et al. Pulmonary hypertension: pulmonary flow quantification and flow profile analysis with velocity-encoded cine MR imaging. Radiology 1992;183(3):751–8.
22. Muthurangu V, Taylor A, Andriantsimiavona R, et al. Novel method of quantifying pulmonary vascular resistance by use of simultaneous invasive pressure monitoring and phase-contrast magnetic resonance flow. Circulation 2004;110(7):826–34.
23. Muthurangu V, Atkinson D, Sermesant M, et al. Measurement of total pulmonary arterial compliance using invasive pressure monitoring and MR flow quantification during MR-guided cardiac catheterization. Am J Physiol Heart Circ Physiol 2005;289(3):H1301–6.
24. Rhode KS, Hill DL, Edwards PJ, et al. Registration and tracking to integrate X-ray and MR images in an XMR facility. IEEE Trans Med Imaging 2003;22(11):1369–78.
25. Razavi RS, Baker A, Qureshi SA, et al. Hemodynamic response to continuous infusion of dobutamine in Alagille's syndrome. Transplantation 2001;72(5):823–8.
26. Bakker CJ, Hoogeveen RM, Weber J, et al. Visualization of dedicated catheters using fast scanning techniques with potential for MR-guided vascular interventions. Magn Reson Med 1996;36(6):816–20.
27. Bakker CJ, Smits HF, Bos C, et al. MR-guided balloon angioplasty: in vitro demonstration of the potential of MRI for guiding, monitoring, and evaluating endovascular interventions. J Magn Reson Imaging 1998;8(1):245–50.

28. Bakker CJ, Bos C, Weinmann HJ. Passive tracking of catheters and guidewires by contrast-enhanced MR fluoroscopy. Magn Reson Med 2001;45(1):17–23.

29. Bakker CJ, Hoogeveen RM, Hurtak WF, et al. MR-guided endovascular interventions: susceptibility-based catheter and near-real-time imaging technique. Radiology 1997;202(1):273–6.

30. Dumoulin CL, Souza SP, Darrow RD. Real-time position monitoring of invasive devices using magnetic resonance. Magn Reson Med 1993;29(3):411–5.

31. Ladd ME, Zimmermann GG, McKinnon GC, et al. Visualization of vascular guidewires using MR tracking. J Magn Reson Imaging 1998;8(1):251–3.

32. Ladd ME, Zimmermann GG, Quick HH, et al. Active MR visualization of a vascular guidewire in vivo. J Magn Reson Imaging 1998;8(1):220–5.

33. Ladd ME, Quick HH. Reduction of resonant RF heating in intravascular catheters using coaxial chokes. Magn Reson Med 2000;43(4):615–9.

34. Zhang Q, Wendt M, Aschoff AJ, et al. Active MR guidance of interventional devices with target-navigation. Magn Reson Med 2000;44(1):56–65.

35. Hillenbrand CM, Elgort DR, Wong EY, et al. Active device tracking and high-resolution intravascular MRI using a novel catheter-based, opposed-solenoid phased array coil. Magn Reson Med 2004; 51(4):668–75.

36. Glowinski A, Adam G, Bucker A, et al. Catheter visualization using locally induced, actively controlled field inhomogeneities. Magn Reson Med 1997; 38(2):253–8.

37. Konings MK, Bartels LW, Smits HF, et al. Heating around intravascular guidewires by resonating RF waves. J Magn Reson Imaging 2000;12:79–85.

38. Weiss S, Vernickel P, Schaeffter T, et al. Transmission line for improved RF safety of interventional devices. Magn Reson Med 2005;54:182–9.

39. Weiss S, Kuehne T, Brinkert F, et al. In vivo safe catheter visualization and slice tracking using an optically detunable resonant marker. Magn Reson Med 2004;52:860–8.

40. Hegde S, Miquel ME, Boubertakh R, et al. Interactive MR imaging and tracking of catheters with multiple tuned fiducial markers. J Vasc Interv Radiol 2006;17:1175–9.

41. Rickers C, Jerosch-Herold M, Hu X, et al. Magnetic resonance image-guided transcatheter closure of atrial septal defects. Circulation 2003;107:132–8.

42. Arepally A, Karmarkar PV, Weiss C, et al. Magnetic resonance image-guided trans-septal puncture in a swine heart. J Magn Reson Imaging 2005;21:463–7.

43. Buecker A, Spuentrup E, Grabitz R, et al. Magnetic resonance-guided placement of atrial septal closure device in animal model of patent foramen ovale. Circulation 2002;106:511–5.

44. Raval AN, Karmarkar PV, Guttman MA, et al. Real-time MRI guided atrial septal puncture and balloon septostomy in swine. Catheter Cardiovasc Interv 2006;67:637–43.

45. Qiu B, Gao F, Karmarkar P, et al. Intracoronary MR imaging using a 0.014-inch MR imaging-guidewire: toward MRI-guided coronary interventions. J Magn Reson Imaging 2008;28:515–8.

46. Serfaty JM, Yang X, Foo TK, et al. MRI-guided coronary catheterization and PTCA: A feasibility study on a dog model. Magn Reson Med 2003;49:258–63.

47. Feng L, Dumoulin CL, Dashnaw S, et al. Feasibility of stent placement in carotid arteries with real-time MR imaging guidance in pigs. Radiology 2005;234: 558–62.

48. Raval AN, Karmarkar PV, Guttman MA, et al. Real-time magnetic resonance imaging-guided endovascular recanalization of chronic total arterial occlusion in a swine model. Circulation 2006;113:1101–7.

49. Kuehne T, Weiss S, Brinkert F, et al. Catheter visualization with resonant markers at MR imaging-guided deployment of endovascular stents in swine. Radiology 2004;233:774–80.

50. Spuentrup E, Ruebben A, Schaeffter T, et al. Magnetic resonance–guided coronary artery stent placement in a swine model. Circulation 2002;105: 874–9.

51. Kuehne T, Saeed M, Higgins CB, et al. Endovascular stents in pulmonary valve and artery in swine: feasibility study of MR imaging-guided deployment and post interventional assessment. Radiology 2003; 226:475–81.

52. Saeed M, Henk CB, Weber O, et al. Delivery and assessment of endovascular stents to repair aortic coarctation using MR and X-ray imaging. J Magn Reson Imaging 2006;24:371–8.

53. Raval AN, Telep JD, Guttman MA, et al. Real-time magnetic resonance imaging-guided stenting of aortic coarctation with commercially available catheter devices in Swine. Circulation 2005;112: 699–706.

54. Arepally A, Karmarkar PV, Qian D, et al. Evaluation of MR/fluoroscopy-guided portosystemic shunt creation in a swine model. J Vasc Interv Radiol 2006; 17:1165–73.

55. Shih MC, Rogers WJ, Hagspiel KD. Real-time magnetic resonance-guided placement of retrievable inferior vena cava filters: comparison with fluoroscopic guidance with use of in vitro and animal models. J Vasc Interv Radiol 2006;17:327–33.

56. Tzifa A, Krombach GA, Krämer N, et al. Magnetic resonance-guided cardiac interventions using magnetic resonance-compatible devices: a preclinical study and first-in-man congenital interventions. Circ Cardiovasc Interv 2010;3(6):585–92.

Postmortem MR Imaging in the Fetal and Neonatal Period

Maarten H. Lequin, MD[a],*,
Thierry A.G.M. Huisman, MD, EQNR, FICIS[b]

KEYWORDS

• Postmortem • MR Imaging • Autopsy • Neonates

Today postmortem imaging has become an increasingly important part of the examination of deceased fetuses and neonates. For centuries postmortem examination consisted only of a classical autopsy, which is still considered to be the gold standard.[1–3] The pathologist's role is to establish the exact cause of death, which is often an important factor in the bereavement process of parents, especially when they are concerned about the correctness of their decisions during pregnancy.[1,2,4–6] However, identification of the reason for fetal and neonatal death serves many more important goals. Autopsy results are also of great value for genetic counseling, not only for assessing the recurrence rate of a specific syndrome but also for implementation of strategies for prevention of unnecessary risks in future pregnancies.[4,7] Risk estimation for recurrence may, however, be hampered by parental refusal of autopsy because of religious or philosophic beliefs. In this case, one can only rely on prenatal tests for counseling of future pregnancies. Another important issue is the medicolegal aspect, where postmortem confirmation of the prenatal diagnosis or suspected fetal pathology may validate the performed obstetric strategy. This may relieve both parents and physicians of blame.[1,5] Finally, identification of the exact fetal pathology and cause of death advances medical knowledge by allowing clinicians to monitor and validate therapies, which eventually improves clinical practice and research.[2,4,5]

Notwithstanding the acceptance of the undisputable value of autopsy worldwide, autopsy rates are continuously declining.[2,4,5] Many studies, including those meta-analysis based, show high clinicopathologic discrepancy rates, varying between 22% and 76%.[1–4,8,9] Additionally, one autopsy study shows a change in recurrence risk estimation or parental counseling in more than 26% of cases.[1] Therefore, it is of utmost importance to understand why autopsy rates are declining and, if this process is inevitable, to explore and develop alternative postmortem diagnostic techniques.

The reason for the decline in autopsies is multifactorial and complex.[10,11] The impact of the perception and acceptance by the general public, clinicians, and pathologists of autopsies is significant. The low public consent rate is one of the most important reasons for the observed decline.[10] The consent rate seems to depend on religion, ethnic origin, cultural attitude, media portrayal of autopsies, and public perceptions. Religious and ethnic beliefs may strongly oppose autopsy and anatomic dissection. In addition, the religious necessity that the burial takes place within 24 hours may also interfere with or prevent autopsy.[12] As a result, the fetal or neonatal brain has to be examined unfixed, preventing detailed analysis.[13] Newer agents, such as picric acid and formaldehyde, make an adequate overnight fixation and immersion possible, but the technical limitations of removing the watery, unfixed brain

[a] Department of Pediatric Radiology, Sophia Children's Hospital, University Hospital Rotterdam, Dr Molewaterplein 60, 3015 GJ Rotterdam, The Netherlands
[b] Division of Pediatric Radiology, Department of Radiology and Radiological Science, Johns Hopkins Hospital, 600 North Wolfe Street, Nelson, B-173, Baltimore, MD 21287–0842, USA
* Corresponding author.
E-mail address: m.lequin@erasmusmc.nl

Magn Reson Imaging Clin N Am 20 (2012) 129–143
doi:10.1016/j.mric.2011.08.008

from the cranial vault are still tremendous.[13] With regard to the clinician, the decline in autopsy rate is caused by the time-consuming consent process, the assumption that advances in premortem diagnostic techniques diminish the need for autopsy, and that a grieving family is hostile to the idea of autopsy.[10] For some pathologists autopsy is an unpleasant, time-consuming procedure often regarded as secondary to their primary duties, best delegated to a junior trainee.[14] Also, the lack of communication between the clinician and the pathologist further limits the clinical value of autopsy.

Therefore, there is a continuous need to improve the awareness of the clinical value of autopsy not only for clinicians and pathologists, but also for the public. In addition, alternative postmortem diagnostic procedures have emerged. These include minimally invasive autopsies, such as endoscopic and needle tissue aspiration and autopsy, with or without ultrasonography (US)[15] or computed-tomography (CT) guidance.[16] Endoscopic autopsy has some drawbacks that limit its use. One of them is its need for special equipment and expertise. In addition, several anatomic regions are difficult to reach, such as the posterior mediastinum and retroperitoneum.[17] Needle biopsies or autopsies may be an alternative for complete autopsy, especially if organs are diffusely affected. However, because this technique does not allow for inspection or dissection of the internal organs directly, valuable macroscopic information is lacking. In addition, although needle autopsy may give important information about the cause of death, not all causes for fetal or neonatal fatal outcome can be determined. When there are congenital anomalies, especially cardiovascular abnormalities, minimally invasive autopsies cannot replace conventional autopsies.

Noninvasive postmortem imaging studies, such as conventional radiography, US, CT, and MR imaging, are valuable alternatives and additions to conventional autopsy. Conventional radiography of the deceased child has been an important tool to confirm or reject the antenatal diagnosis for many decades. Especially in children with skeletal dysplasia radiography is still the primary imaging modality. With the introduction of other imaging modalities, such as US, CT, and MR imaging, also known as "virtopsies,"[18] new indications for postmortem imaging have emerged. Of these three cross-sectional imaging modalities, US is the least favored technique, not only because it is operator-dependent and sonographers feel uneasy to examine a deceased fetus or neonate, but most of all it is never possible to

have an overview of all the abnormalities present compared with three-dimensional whole-body imaging techniques, such as CT and MR imaging.[18] CT definitely has an established role in postmortem imaging, but mainly in the somewhat older population. CT is especially helpful in children suspected of battering or in cases of death after severe trauma, including forensic cases.[19,20] The low tissue contrast of CT in small fetuses or neonates limits its use, however, as an alternative for classical autopsy. Postmortem MR imaging or MR autopsy became the best alternative postmortem imaging tool because of its high spatial resolution, excellent contrast and signal-to-noise ratio, and the multitude of image contrasts that can be generated. MR autopsy consequently allows one to better delineate the different tissues of the deceased body.[21]

This article discusses how to perform MR autopsy, including such technical determinators as field strength, and factors influencing image quality, followed by a discussion of the indications for MR autopsy. Also explored are such fetal issues as stillborns and terminations of pregnancy, and postnatal issues of natural death and unexplained death.

HOW TO PERFORM AND INTERPRET POSTMORTEM MR IMAGING

Informed consent has to be obtained from the parents, emphasizing that the examination is noninvasive and that the integrity of the body is respected. Parents should be aware of the possibility to dress their baby, as they like for the burial or cremation, avoiding metallic objects in the clothing. Necklaces and medallions, which may interact with the magnetic field, must be removed before the examination.

Parents should be informed that postmortem MR imaging cannot replace a complete autopsy; that MR imaging is only an alternative, with the major drawback that no tissue samples are obtained; and that consequently no chromosomal, biochemical, histologic, molecular, or microbiologic analyses are possible.

If one proposes postmortem MR imaging, it should be performed as soon as possible after the child is deceased. In the authors' experience, the time frame depends on what the referring physician wants to know. In cases of termination of pregnancy, the physician seeks confirmation of antenatal diagnosis; in most cases this is an anatomic question or syndromal question. In most cases these questions can still be answered after a couple of days. In the case of a late third-trimester stillborn or deceased neonate, imaging should be done immediately, preferably within 24 hours, thereby avoiding refusals of consent because of cultural habits of burial or cremation within 24 hours.[10] Another reason to scan as early as possible is to minimize the influence of maceration and autolysis of tissues within the deceased body, which decreases tissue contrast.[21] This is especially important in cases where there is a suspicion of brain pathology. Several recent reports discuss the value of using diffusion tensor imaging (DTI) in children with severe brain malformation or those who suffered brain trauma (Fig. 1).[22,23] There are no evidence-based data on this subject, but if the authors use diffusion weighted imaging (DWI) or DTI for postmortem brain imaging, they try to perform the examination within 6 hours after death to limit the impact of

postmortem tissue deterioration on the diffusion characteristics.

Huisman[21] suggested a time frame of 72 hours, in which an excellent image quality is guaranteed, especially when the deceased body is immediately cooled at 4°C. In the authors' experience, cooling has some disadvantages because it decreases the T1- and T2-weighted image contrast, which can be especially limiting in the examination of very small fetuses. Petrén-Mallmin and colleagues[24] also showed a decreased T1- and T2-weighted image contrast related to temperature reduction. They found that T1- and T2-relaxation times of fat tissue decrease almost linearly with decreasing temperature. For other tissues, such as muscle, T1- and T2-relaxation times drop slightly to moderately. Also T2-relaxation time and signal

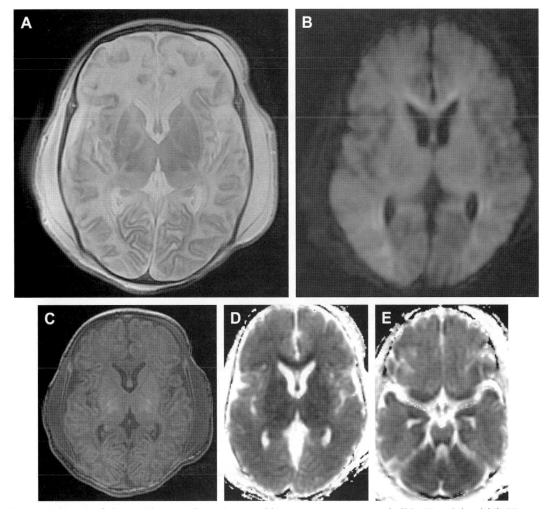

Fig. 1. Multiorgan failure with severe hypoxia caused by pneumococcus encephalitis. T2-weighted (A), T2 trace map (B), T1-weighted image (C), and two ADC maps (D, E). Note restricted diffusion on the ADC maps at the level of the cerebellum, hippocampus, basal ganglia, thalamus, and large parts of the cortex.

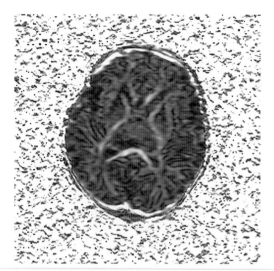

Fig. 2. Fractional anisotropy map of a postmortem brain of a 4-day-old term baby as part of a post-mortem MR imaging examination within 1 hour after unsuccessful reanimation. Fractional anisotropy maps can be used for tractography and for assessment of the brain architecture even postmortem.

intensity of fat and bone marrow show a significant decrease between 37°C and 10 to 20°C, the temperature frame in which the deceased body is scanned.[24] This is important to know because most of the time imaging relies on the T2-weighted sequences because they render high spatial resolution images with optimal contrast between different tissues.

Most postmortem MR imaging is performed on 1.5-T scanners because of their wide availability.[13,25] Because of the recent introduction of clinical 3-T scanners, more experience is gained with this higher field strength but no systematic studies comparing both field strengths have been published. A recently published study showed that ultra-high-field systems, up to 9.4 T, can be used for fetal postmortem imaging.[26]

The selection of the coils depends on the size of the object. In fetuses, phased-array surface coils can be used; in neonates, the circular knee coil or phased-array head coil are available.

In most reports the imaging protocol consists of fast spin-echo T2 sequences in three orthogonal planes. The slice thickness depends on the body size and the area of highest interest. The slice thickness should not exceed 3 mm if the neonatal brain and spine are imaged. For the neonatal thorax and abdomen a slice thickness of 5 mm is sufficient. An imaging matrix of 512 × 512 is optimal, but a 256 × 256 matrix will also do in most cases. Depending on the body size the smallest field-of-view should be chosen. In most cases the entire fetus or neonate is imaged, although coverage of the extremities is not performed routinely. In some cases, after thorough consultation with the referring physician, limited studies of only the brain can be considered. In the authors' experience the number of signal averages should be at least three to optimize the signal-to-noise ratio for diagnostic study quality. The overall scan time normally ranges between 30 and 60 minutes.

In some reports additional T2 spin density weighted sequence is suggested to increase the contrast between cerebral gray and white matter. The use of DWI/DTI for the brain can be performed in selected cases (**Fig. 2**). The b-value should be 1000 s/mm^2 in case of a neonate but should

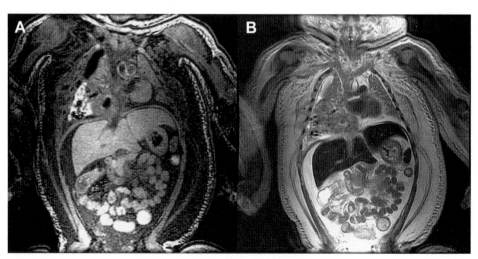

Fig. 3. Coronal T1-weighted image (*A*) shows better the hemorrhagic component of the pneumococcus pneumonia in the right lower lobe compared with the T2-weighted image (*B*).

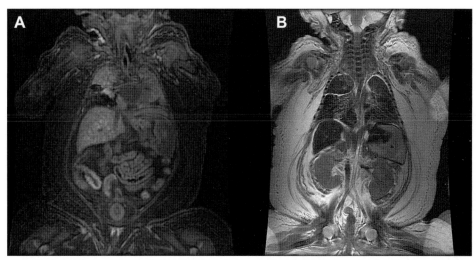

Fig. 4. Coronal T1-weighted image (*A*) delineates better the involvement of the liver and the spleen in this premature infant with *Klebsiella* sepsis compared with the T2-weighted image (*B*). Note also the assessment of destruction of the right lower lobe.

be adjusted to the gestational age in younger babies. Like Breeze and colleagues,[27] many experts in postmortem MR imaging believe that T1-weighted sequences add little valuable information. In the authors' experience the three-dimensional T1 gradient echo sequence may have some advantages. First, postprocessing of the three-dimensional data set allows correcting for position differences between different parts of the body because of rigor. Second, the possibility of three-dimensional interpretation and maximum intensity projection may be helpful for reading out. Finally, T1 information of structures and focal lesions (eg, hemorrhages, meconium, and calcifications) is also obtained. This could be of help in a detailed evaluation and localization of focal pathologies in the brain, such as differentiating between germinal matrix or bleeding. In the chest T1-weighted sequences may also help to diagnose pneumonia much easier than on T2-weighted images (**Fig. 3**). In the abdomen, liver disease is sometimes better seen on T1-weighted images (**Fig. 4**), and meconium content in the bowel is better seen on T1- than on T2-weighted images because of the high T1-signal of meconium.

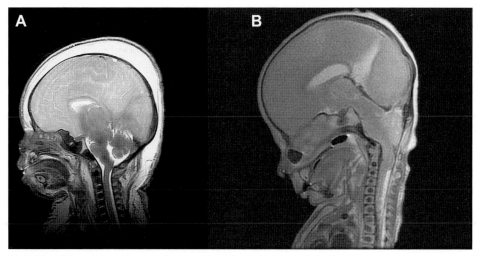

Fig. 5. (*A*) Sagittal T2-weighted image shows a physiologic kinking of the brainstem as a postmortem effect on the left. (*B*) On the right an example of a Chiari type 2 malformation with kinking of the craniocervical junction and tonsillar herniation at the level of C2.

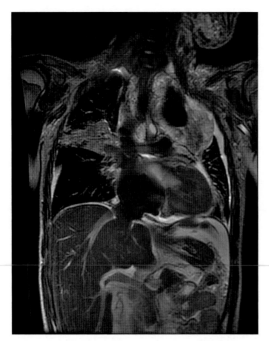

Fig. 6. Coronal T2-weighted image shows a clot in the right pulmonary artery. This may be a postmortem effect, but in this case it also resulted in a lung infarct of the basal part of the right upper lobe. Note the lymphangioma in the neck on the left, extending in the thorax and mediastinum.

Image interpretation should be done or supervised by an experienced pediatric (neuro) radiologist who is familiar with fetal anatomy, embryology, and pathology. In the optimal setting, the evaluation of

the images should be done within a multidisciplinary team, including obstetricians (preferable the one who performed the antenatal ultrasounds); pediatricians; pediatric neurologists; geneticists; and pathologists. Some reports even suggest the creation of a new subspecialty: postmortem radiology or necroradiology. This seems to be especially valuable in forensic cases.[28]

In the authors' practice, the referring partners are consulted for interpretation in most cases but frequently (>60%) no complete autopsy has been performed, leaving out the consultation of the pathologist to save time for the radiologist or pathologist. This seems to be a suboptimal procedure, because previous studies show an improvement in diagnostic accuracy of fetal anomalies after autopsy, using protocol-based investigation, report, and interdisciplinary consultation in cases of termination of pregnancy. This is especially true in situations with multiple congenital abnormalities, including cardiac malformations.

The best start is to follow a standardized reading protocol. The report should include dedicated sections on the brain and spine, neck and thorax, abdomen, and skeleton as far as it was included in the imaging protocol.

The major point that should always be kept in mind is that postmortem imaging is not simply the same as clinical imaging of a living child.[28] Because of lack of cardiac output, intravenous contrast administration is not possible. This makes interpretation of the thoracic cavity including the heart more problematic. Also, the lack of blood

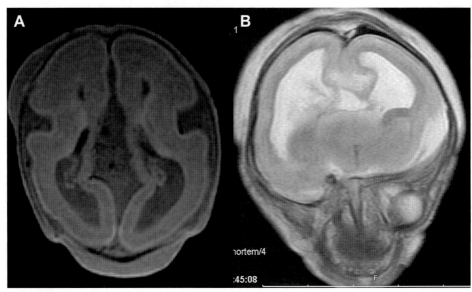

Fig. 7. (*A*) Axial T1-weighted image of a 23-week-old fetus with a classical callosal agenesis. (*B*) Coronal T2-weighted image delineates the fusion of the thalamus as part of a semilobar holoprosencephaly in a 17-week-old fetus.

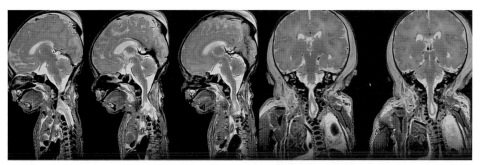

Fig. 8. Sagittal and coronal T2-weighted images showing an example of a neuroenteric fistula with spinal abnormalities.

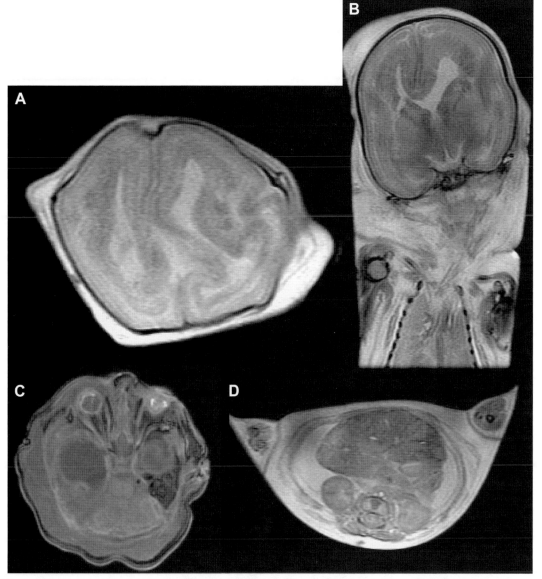

Fig. 9. (*A, B*) Axial and coronal T2-weighted images of a 21-week-old fetus show a migration disorder, periventricular located, with low signal intensity compatible with calcifications caused by toxoplasmosis. (*C*) Axial T1-weighted image of the bulbus oculi demonstrates high signal intensity, representing chorioretinitis. (*D*) Axial T2-weighted image of the liver shows a small liver, inhomogeneous signal intensity with low signal caused by calcifications and infiltrates of toxoplasmosis. Note also ascites.

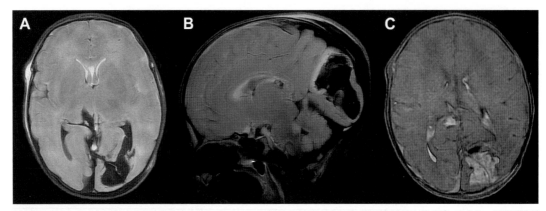

Fig. 10. Axial and sagittal T2-weighted (*A*, *B*) and axial T1-weighted images (*C*) show the direction of the knife stab through the belly of a pregnant woman into the left occipital lobe of a 38-week-old fetus. Note the laceration of the sinus rectus and damage to the right posteromedial part of the thalamus.

pressure can change the shape of the anatomy dramatically, not only in vessels but also in the brain, resulting in a physiologic kinking of the brain stem in the posterior fossa, which should not be interpreted as a Chiari malformation (**Fig. 5**). Moreover, after death blood elements sediment out, a process known as "lividity,"[29] and intravascular clots can occur (**Fig. 6**). Also, gas formation may be seen because of putrefaction, which should not be misinterpreted as free air or portal air. To minimize these artifacts, postmortem MR imaging should be performed immediately after death. Another point is that, particularly in forensic cases, it is possible to see signs of disease or the presence of foreign bodies, rarely detected in the living, but frequently seen by pathologists.

Finally, recent reports show that higher field strengths give a greater spatial resolution, higher tissue contrast, and better diagnostic information. Especially in a fetus less than 20 weeks of gestation ultra-high-field MR imaging (>7 T) has advantages compared with conventional 1.5-T imaging.[26] Ultra-high-field MR imaging increases the diagnostic usefulness of postmortem imaging because of the possibility of creating thin-sliced isotropic three-dimensional images within a clinically acceptable scan time. Therefore, a better agreement with autopsy findings results particularly in the area where 1.5-T imaging has a low agreement concordance, especially in the brain, spinal cord, and heart. A disadvantage of ultra-high-field imaging may be the possible increase of positive findings that are not confirmed or remain undetected at autopsy.

Future research has to be performed to assess the value and significance of these positive findings noticed not only on ultra high field MR imaging

but also on 1.5-T MR imaging for parental counseling.

POSTMORTEM MR IMAGING INDICATIONS
Fetal Indications

Most fetal imaging is done on second-trimester fetuses, mainly because in this period the obstetrician or prenatal interdisciplinary team (in combination with the parents) makes the decision of terminating pregnancy. In second-trimester fetuses, most abnormalities are developmental and often have obvious macroscopic manifestations, which can easily be classified by postmortem MR imaging. Examples include pathologies of the kidneys; liver; gut; abdominal wall (gastroschisis, omphalocele); and central nervous system (corpus callosum agenesis, holoprosencephaly, spinal dysraphia) (**Fig. 7**). In the authors' practice, the focus is on suspected abnormalities of the brain and spinal cord (**Fig. 8**) because this area may be difficult to assess with antenatal US. Migrational abnormalities, impaired cortical organization, abnormal myelinization of the white matter, or complex malformations, such as Aicardi syndrome and muscle-eye-brain disease, or metabolic disorders, such as Zellweger syndrome, are difficult to diagnose in complete detail prenatally. Other body parts are in most cases easier to screen by antenatal US. Another reason for focusing on the brain with MR imaging is the difficulty of preservation and handling of the fetal brain by the (neuro) pathologist because of maceration and small head size, resulting in a 20% failure rate in autopsy studies.[30,31] Also the investigation of the spinal cord is difficult for the pathologist because the small, immature spinal cord is frequently damaged during removal from the bony spinal canal.[11] This low overall contribution of histologic examination

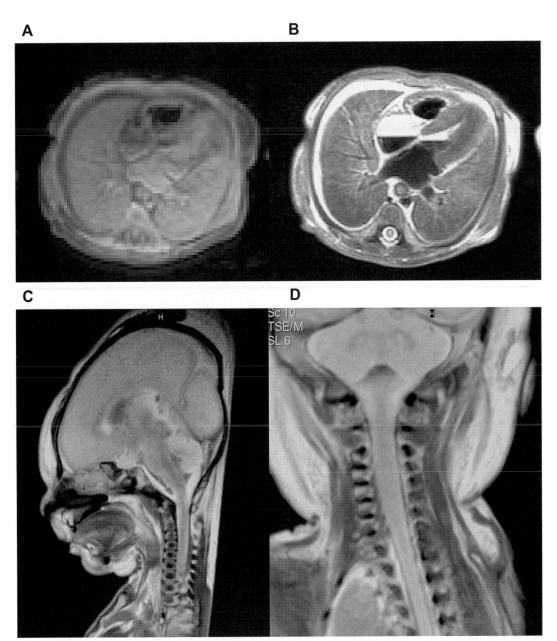

Fig. 11. Acute arrest in a 27-week premature fetus after flushing intravenous catheter. (*A*) Note air in right ventricle best seen on this T1-weighted image. (*B*) On the T2-weighted image differentiating between fresh blood products and air may be difficult. Sagittal (*C*) and coronal (*D*) images showing a transsection at the level of the brainstem with hemorrhage and at the level of the cervical myelum caused by severe birth trauma. Note the severe swelling of the spinal cord at this level.

in congenital abnormalities of the central nervous system cases is a major limitation of conventional autopsy, considering that the central nervous system is the most frequently involved "organ" that is malformed.[32] The overall incidence is about 1% of live births and even higher in terminations of pregnancy.[32] Therefore, postmortem MR imaging may be the best technique to assess central nervous system abnormalities in a very small fetus, even when a significant degree of maceration is present.[7] In the authors' practice the pathologist is even in some cases the referring doctor to ask for a postmortem MR imaging of the brain before full autopsy.

Postmortem MR imaging has its limitations for some areas of the body. In particular the heart is a difficult region because of the altered shape

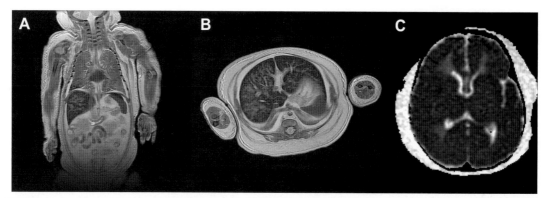

Fig. 12. Coronal and axial T2-weighted images delineating lung, but especially liver involvement in a 23-week-old fetus with herpes simplex type 2 infection. (*A*) Note the patchy involvement of the liver caused by infiltration of herpes virus and small infarcts. The signal around these areas is still normal. (*B*) The spleen looks spared, although it has slightly higher signal intensity than normal. No splenic infarcts. Ascites and periportal fluid. (*C*) Coronal ADC map demonstrates total brain asphyxia caused by sepsis.

and anatomy after decease, because no blood flow and pressure are present to expand the heart. In addition, no dynamic flow data are present, which may prevent identification of functional disorders, such as an insufficient cardiac valve or reversed blood flow direction. Woodward and coworkers[33] and Alderliesten and colleagues[7] mention limitations in evaluating discrete anomalous connections between anatomic structures and exact identification of skeletal malformations. This may be partially solved by performing ultra-high-field MR imaging; however, postmortem MR imaging never gives functional and dynamic data.

In the third trimester fetus and stillborn child matters may become more complicated because of a higher rate of acquired diseases resulting in death. One has to think of hypoxic, ischemic, or hemorrhagic events, and intrauterine infections (**Fig. 9**). The correct differentiation between an acquired pathology and possibly inherited malformation is essential for counseling. In many cases, histologic confirmation remains valuable but in some cases imaging may be diagnostic or may suggest the diagnosis, which for example could be tested by microbiologic analyses or needle biopsy if there was no consent to conventional autopsy.

Finally, cases of nonnatural fetal death caused by a car accident or other trauma, such as stab wounds inflicted to the mother during pregnancy (**Fig. 10**), could be an indication for postmortem MR imaging for medicolegal purposes. Furthermore, postmortem imaging may give a better three-dimensional image especially in view of stab wounds, revealing how and in which direction the stabbing occurred and which organs were injured without disrupting the anatomy because of dissection or removal of organs in case of autopsy.

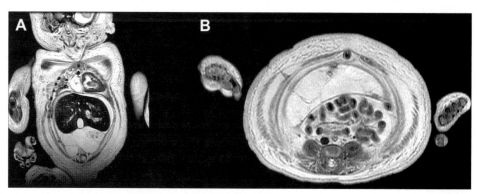

Fig. 13. Coronal and axial T2-weighted images of a 31-week-old premature infant with unexplained hydrops fetalis. (*A*) Note the edema of the skin, muscles, and subcutaneous fat. (*B*) Because of the presence of intrathoracic and intra-abdominal lymphangiomas the diagnosis of Hennekam syndrome was made.

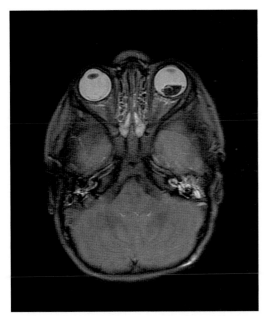

Fig. 14. Axial T2-weighted image showing a low signal in the left bulbus oculi caused by retinal bleeding in a 3-week-old infant suspected for battering. Note also the severe brain swelling in the posterior fossa, obliterating the fourth ventricle and pushing the brainstem into the clivus.

Neonatal Indications

In the neonatal period the indications to perform postmortem MR imaging include iatrogenic or birth-related causes of death (**Fig. 11**). Also, severe infections resulting in sepsis and multiorgan failure may be an indication for postmortem MR imaging (eg, neonatal herpes simplex infection), especially to rule out other causes of neonatal death (**Fig. 12**). Unexplained hydrops fetalis or severe respiratory distress followed by death belongs to these indications (**Fig. 13**). Postmortem MR imaging is especially helpful in cases of suspected nonaccidental injury including shaken baby syndrome, in which the brain can be examined in the cranial vault without additional injury related to the removal of the brain for autopsy. Although more frequently seen in older children, battering does occur in the neonatal period (**Fig. 14**). In addition, postmortem MR imaging should be considered if imaging studies before neonatal death do not explain the clinical course. Postmortem MR imaging could show subtle findings that remained undetected during life. Frequently, the neonate is too unstable to be moved to the MR imaging suite for examination and consequently the initial imaging is limited to head ultrasound studies or fast CT examinations. In addition, advanced MR imaging techniques, such as ^1H magnetic resonance spectroscopy, may identify metabolic disease (eg, nonketotic hyperglycinemia) that remained undetected on conventional imaging (**Fig. 15** and **Table 1**).[34] A complete autopsy remains the gold standard, but MR autopsy can be a helpful alternative or complementing technique.

LIMITATIONS OF POSTMORTEM MR IMAGING?

Postmortem MR imaging cannot currently replace full autopsy, but it has definitely a role, especially in cases when autopsy is not consented to by the parents or caregivers. Postmortem MR imaging is very sensitive to detect abnormalities, but the specificity is low. The radiologist and referring physicians should be aware of the strengths but

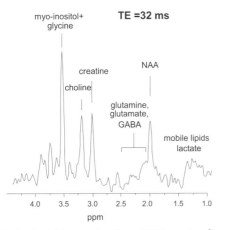

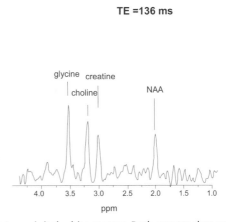

Fig. 15. Short and long echo time PRESS spectra from parieto-occipital white matter. Both spectra demonstrate the high intensity of glycine in the brain at 3.6 ppm. GABA, gamma-aminobutyric acid; NAA, *N*-acetyl aspartate.

Table 1 Concentration of glycine in different regions of the brain		
Brain Region	**Quantitative** **¹H MR** **Spectroscopy[a]** **mmol/L**	**Chemical** **Quantification[b]** **mmol/L**
Cerebrospinal fluid	<1	0.46
Occipito-parietal white matter	4 ± 0.3	4.24
Frontal white matter	5 ± 0.5	4.86
Basal ganglia	5.5 ± 0.5	6.61
Cerebellar white matter	8 ± 0.7	(not available)

[a] Study done on postnatal day 7.
[b] Study done at postnatal day 9, 12 hours postmortem.

also the limitations of postmortem MR imaging. The most frequently reported discrepancies compared with autopsy are discussed next for the different anatomic regions.

Brain

For the brain, MR imaging is comparable or even superior to autopsy in most cases.[7,11,21,27] In prenatally induced feticide, frequently performed to reduce the head circumference in fetuses with congenital hydrocephalus to facilitate delivery, the fetal brain can be severely distorted making interpretation very difficult (**Fig. 16**). When using a 1.5-T MR imaging unit, assessment of the brain parenchyma may be difficult because of a low signal-to-noise ratio in very small fetuses. Only centers with high- or ultra-high-field scanners may overcome this problem.[26]

Neck and Thorax

In contrast to prenatal MR imaging the trachea and esophagus are not filled with fluid, making

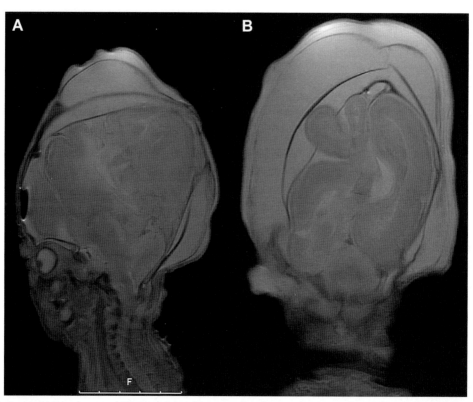

Fig. 16. Sagittal (*A*) and coronal (*B*) T2-weighted images after brain puncture to facilitate labor. Interpretation of these images is hampered.

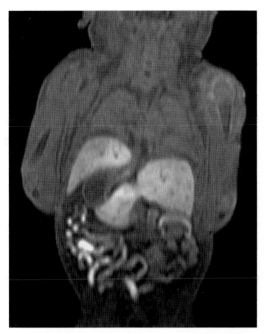

Fig. 17. Coronal reconstructed image of a three-dimensional T1-weighted sequence demonstrates an ambiguous position of the liver, stomach on the right site. Asplenia and malposition of the intestinals, hyperintens colon caused by meconium is positioned in the right side of the abdomen.

the diagnosis of tracheal and esophageal atresia or fistula very challenging.[27] Diagnosing lung hypoplasia is in most cases possible but exact assessment of the pulmonary lobulation is nearly impossible.[27] Abnormal MR imaging signal intensity of the lung parenchyma may not have a matching underlying histopathology.[27]

Heart and Vessels

This is by far the most difficult area to evaluate. Cardiac atria and ventricles are distinguishable but septa and outflow tracts are difficult to assess. Three-dimensional MR imaging techniques, particularly in the case of ultra-high-field MR scanning, may help but autopsy still remains the gold standard. Coarctation of the aorta may be missed on postmortem MR imaging.[7] Thrombus formation in the pulmonary arteries may be a postmortem effect instead of the major cause of death.

Abdomen

Bowel rotation or atresia may be difficult to detect (**Fig. 17**). Alderliesten and colleagues[7] also mentioned problems with abdominal wall defects and anus atresia, but these abnormalities are usually obvious on physical examination. Most organs are well delineated on MR imaging; however, depiction of the pancreas may be difficult on T2-weighted images.T1-weighted images have proved to be helpful for the evaluation of the pancreas (**Fig. 18**).

Skeleton

Frequently, only part of the skeleton is included in the field of view. Consequently, a correct overall diagnosis of skeletal dysplasia is difficult to make (**Fig. 19**). Malformations of the extremities are usually better examined by visual inspection in combination with conventional radiography.

FUTURE OF POSTMORTEM MR IMAGING

It is still a bridge to far to say that postmortem MR imaging with or without image-guided additional fine-needle biopsy could replace full autopsy. It should, however, be considered as a valuable alternative tool if parents refuse conventional autopsy. With ongoing hardware (higher field strengths) and software developments (tissue-specific imaging sequences) postmortem MR imaging may play a bigger role in the postmortem evaluation of fetuses and neonates in the near

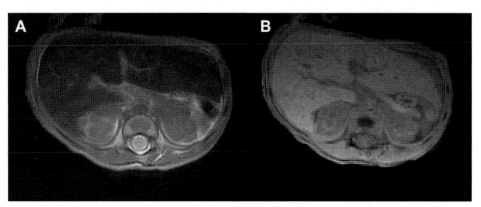

Fig. 18. Axial T2-weighted (*A*) and T1-weighted (*B*) images better delineate the pancreas on the latter image.

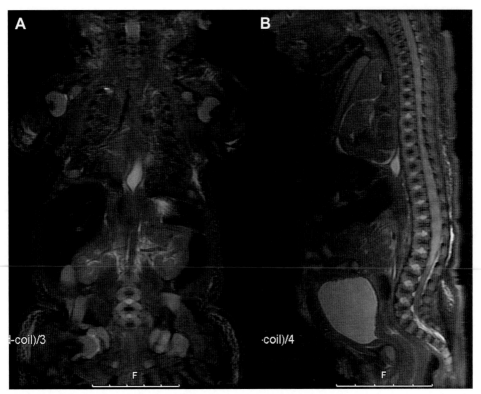

Fig. 19. Coronal (*A*) and sagittal (*B*) T2-weighted images show short limbs, abnormal vertebra, and small thoracic shape, all compatible with the diagnosis of thanatrophic dysplasia.

future. The development of age-specific MR imaging parameters, enhancing tissue contrast, may increase the confidence level of reporting abnormalities, particularly in the brain. Advanced MR imaging techniques, such as ¹H MR spectroscopy, may help to identify metabolic diseases noninvasively. Until now, the focus of ¹H MR spectroscopy has been on the brain, but in the future ¹H MR spectroscopy may help to identify metabolic diseases affecting the liver, heart, or bone marrow.

DWI and DTI are already used for postmortem imaging of the brain, including evaluation of the detailed neuroarchitecture of fiber tracts taking advantage of postprocessing techniques, such as tractography. DWI and DTI may also be used for tissue characterization of various other organs and tissues. Thali and colleagues[35] suggested that MR microscopy may be an alternative to postmortem histologic examination. However, this technique has not been implemented into routine practice.

SUMMARY

Clinicians and pathologists should be aware of the possibilities of postmortem MR imaging in fetuses and neonates as a noninvasive alternative to classical autopsy, particularly if the parents refuse a full autopsy. The MR imaging findings should be discussed and evaluated by an interdisciplinary team. To be an important member of this team, the radiologist and their organization must recognize the subspecialty of postmortem radiology and provide a forum to advance scientific knowledge in the field.

REFERENCES

1. Faye-Petersen OM, Guinn DA, Wenstrom KD. Value of perinatal autopsy. Obstet Gynecol 1999;94(6): 915–20.
2. Kumar P, Angst DB, Taxy J, et al. Neonatal autopsies: a 10-year experience. Arch Pediatr Adolesc Med 2000;154(1):38–42.
3. Gordijn SJ, Erwich JJ, Khong TY. Value of the perinatal autopsy: critique. Pediatr Dev Pathol 2002; 5(5):480–8.
4. Brodlie M, Laing IA, Keeling JW, et al. Ten years of neonatal autopsies in tertiary referral centre: retrospective study. BMJ 2002;324(7340):761–3.
5. Okah FA. The autopsy: experience of a regional neonatal intensive care unit. Paediatr Perinat Epidemiol 2002;16(4):350–4.

6. Wright C, Fenton A, Embleton N. Neonatal necropsy. Lancet 2001;357(9262):1128.

7. Alderliesten ME, Peringa J, van der Hulst VP, et al. Perinatal mortality: clinical value of postmortem magnetic resonance imaging compared with autopsy in routine obstetric practice. BJOG 2003;110(4):378–82.

8. Barr P, Hunt R. An evaluation of the autopsy following death in a level IV neonatal intensive care unit. J Paediatr Child Health 1999;35(2):185–9.

9. Tavora F, Crowder CD, Sun CC, et al. Discrepancies between clinical and autopsy diagnoses: a comparison of university, community, and private autopsy practices. Am J Clin Pathol 2008;129(1):102–9.

10. Burton JL, Underwood J. Clinical, educational, and epidemiological value of autopsy. Lancet 2007; 369(9571):1471–80.

11. Griffiths PD, Paley MN, Whitby EH. Post-mortem MRI as an adjunct to fetal or neonatal autopsy. Lancet 2005;365(9466):1271–3.

12. Sheikh A. Death and dying: a Muslim perspective. J R Soc Med 1998;91(3):138–40.

13. Griffiths PD, Variend D, Evans M, et al. Postmortem MR imaging of the fetal and stillborn central nervous system. AJNR Am J Neuroradiol 2003;24(1):22–7.

14. Bayer-Garner IB, Fink LM, Lamps LW. Pathologists in a teaching institution assess the value of the autopsy. Arch Pathol Lab Med 2002;126(4):442–7.

15. Farina J, Millana C, Fdez-Acenero MJ, et al. Ultrasonographic autopsy (echopsy): a new autopsy technique. Virchows Arch 2002;440(6):635–9.

16. Aghayev E, Ebert LC, Christe A, et al. CT data-based navigation for post-mortem biopsy: a feasibility study. J Forensic Leg Med 2008;15(6):382–7.

17. Avrahami R, Watemberg S, Daniels-Philips E, et al. Endoscopic autopsy. Am J Forensic Med Pathol 1995;16(2):147–50.

18. Uchigasaki S, Oesterhelweg L, Gehl A, et al. Application of compact ultrasound imaging device to postmortem diagnosis. Forensic Sci Int 2004; 140(1):33–41.

19. Flodmark O, Becker LE, Harwood-Nash DC, et al. Correlation between computed tomography and autopsy in premature and full-term neonates that have suffered perinatal asphyxia. Radiology 1980; 137(1 Pt 1):93–103.

20. Stein KM, Grunberg K. Forensic radiology. Radiologe 2009;49(1):73–84 [quiz: 85] [in German].

21. Huisman TA. Magnetic resonance imaging: an alternative to autopsy in neonatal death? Semin Neonatol 2004;9(4):347–53.

22. Widjaja E, Geibprasert S, Blaser S, et al. Abnormal fetal cerebral laminar organization in cobblestone complex as seen on post-mortem MRI and DTI. Pediatr Radiol 2009;39(8):860–4.

23. Watanabe T, Honda Y, Fujii Y, et al. Serial evaluation of axonal function in patients with brain death by using anisotropic diffusion-weighted magnetic resonance imaging. J Neurosurg 2004;100(1): 56–60.

24. Petrén-Mallmin M, Ericsson A, Rauschning W, et al. The effect of temperature on MR relaxation times and signal intensities for human tissues. MAGMA 1993;1(3–4):176–84.

25. Huisman TA, Wisser J, Stallmach T, et al. MR autopsy in fetuses. Fetal Diagn Ther 2002;17(1): 58–64.

26. Thayyil S, Cleary JO, Sebire NJ, et al. Post-mortem examination of human fetuses: a comparison of whole-body high-field MRI at 9.4 T with conventional MRI and invasive autopsy. Lancet 2009;374(9688): 467–75.

27. Breeze AC, Cross JJ, Hackett GA, et al. Use of a confidence scale in reporting postmortem fetal magnetic resonance imaging. Ultrasound Obstet Gynecol 2006;28(7):918–24.

28. O'Donnell C, Woodford N. Post-mortem radiology: a new sub-specialty? Clin Radiol 2008;63(11): 1189–94.

29. Jackowski C, Schweitzer W, Thali M, et al. Virtopsy: postmortem imaging of the human heart in situ using MSCT and MRI. Forensic Sci Int 2005;149(1):11–23.

30. Cartlidge PH, Dawson AT, Stewart JH, et al. Value and quality of perinatal and infant postmortem examinations: cohort analysis of 400 consecutive deaths. BMJ 1995;310(6973):155–8.

31. Vujanic GM, Cartlidge PH, Stewart JH, et al. Perinatal and infant postmortem examinations: how well are we doing? J Clin Pathol 1995;48(11):998–1001.

32. Pinar H, Tatevosyants N, Singer DB. Central nervous system malformations in a perinatal/neonatal autopsy series. Pediatr Dev Pathol 1998;1(1):42–8.

33. Woodward PJ, Sohaey R, Harris DP, et al. Postmortem fetal MR imaging: comparison with findings at autopsy. AJR Am J Roentgenol 1997;168(1): 41–6.

34. Huisman TA, Thiel T, Steinmann B, et al. Proton magnetic resonance spectroscopy of the brain of a neonate with nonketotic hyperglycinemia: in vivo-in vitro (ex vivo) correlation. Eur Radiol 2002;12(4): 858–61.

35. Thali MJ, Dirnhofer R, Becker R, et al. Is 'virtual histology' the next step after the 'virtual autopsy'? Magnetic resonance microscopy in forensic medicine. Magn Reson Imaging 2004;22(8):1131–8.

Index

Note: Page numbers of article titles are in **boldface** type.

Magn Reson Imaging Clin N Am 20 (2012) 145–147
doi:10.1016/S1064-9689(11)00126-7
1064-9689/12/$ – see front matter © 2012 Elsevier Inc. All rights reserved.

mri.theclinics.com